HANDBOOK
ON HUMAN NUTRITIONAL
REQUIREMENTS

First printing 1974
Second printing 1975

FAO Nutritional Studies
WHO Monograph Series

No. 28
No. 61

HANDBOOK
ON HUMAN NUTRITIONAL
REQUIREMENTS

R. PASSMORE

Reader in Physiology
University Medical School
Edinburgh, Scotland

B.M. NICOL

Formerly Deputy Director
Nutrition Division
FAO, Rome, Italy

M. NARAYANA RAO

Nutrition Officer
Food Policy
and Nutrition Division
FAO, Rome, Italy

in collaboration with

G.H. BEATON

Professor and Head
Department of Nutrition
School of Hygiene
University of Toronto, Canada

E.M. DEMAYER

Medical Officer
Nutrition, WHO
Geneva, Switzerland

Published by
FAO and WHO

FOOD AND AGRICULTURE ORGANIZATION OF THE UNITED NATIONS
ROME 1974

FOREWORD

The Food and Agriculture Organization of the United Nations (FAO) provides advice and assistance to member governments in their agricultural planning and development so as to ensure that their food supply meets the needs of the people. The World Health Organization (WHO) is concerned with the prevention of disease and the promotion of health. There are in the world many millions of poor persons, among them children, whose health especially suffers because of an insufficiency of the right kind of foods. On the other hand, there are diseases, common among prosperous people, which are associated with dietary excesses. The incidence of some of these diseases has increased in recent years, reaching epidemic proportions in many of the prosperous countries of the world.

For these reasons both FAO and WHO have been concerned with gathering statements on human nutritional requirements — as accurate and generally acceptable as possible — that will provide a sound scientific basis for the programmes and policies of their member governments. In the last twenty years the two organizations have convened eight meetings of Expert Groups, which have reported on energy requirements (calories) and the following essential nutrients: protein, vitamin A, vitamin D, ascorbic acid (vitamin C), thiamine, niacin, riboflavine, folates, cyanocobalamin (vitamin B_{12}), calcium, and iron. The texts of these reports run to hundreds of pages and contain much technical biochemistry, physiology, and clinical medicine. They are also concerned with the epidemiology of deficiency diseases and the ecology of man in relation to his food supply. Hence, the full reports are not easy reading for those whose knowledge of these subjects is limited. This handbook sets forth the specific recommendations for nutrient intakes made by these Expert Groups and aims to provide a commentary written in a language that is intended to be more readily understandable to food administrators, agricultural planners, and applied nutritionists. It is also hoped that this handbook will prove useful to teachers in secondary

schools and colleges and to everyone concerned with health education.

The main task of correlating the reports of the meetings and
of drafting this handbook was undertaken by Dr. R. Passmore,
Mrs. D.L. Bocobo, Dr. B.M. Nicol and Dr. M. Narayana Rao — the
latter two taking especial responsibility for the chapters on energy,
proteins, iron, iodine, fluorine, and other trace elements. A first
draft of the book was reviewed by Dr. G.H. Beaton and Dr. E.M.
DeMaeyer, who made many valuable comments and suggestions
which were taken into account in the preparation of the final
version.

CONTENTS

1. RECOMMENDED INTAKES OF ENERGY AND NUTRIENTS

Foods supply the body with energy in the form of carbohydrate, fat, and protein; the alcohol in beers, wines, and spirits may also be utilized as a source of energy. Foods also provide the body with such materials as amino acids, vitamins, and minerals — all of which are needed for growth and for the maintenance of cells and tissue. Table 1 gives the recommended intakes of energy and eleven nutrients proposed by the FAO/WHO Expert Groups. The text of this handbook indicates for each nutrient the main foods in which it may be found and the effects on health which are likely to result from a deficiency or an excess of the nutrient. There are many other essential nutrients which the diet must supply, but these are present in ample amounts in all common diets. This text does, however, include brief notes on iodine and fluorine, since an insufficient intake of each of these elements is an important cause of ill health.

The recommended intakes are intended for the use of planners. With the aid of tables giving the composition of foods, the recommended intakes of nutrients can be converted into recommendations for average intakes of foods according to age, sex, and physiological status. Then, the total population figure of a country, together with the distribution of the population by age groups and sex, can be used to make estimates of the total national food requirements. Thus the FAO/WHO recommended intakes of nutrients serve as guides for government officials and others whose duty it is to plan agricultural production and to control imports and exports of food, in order to ensure that the food supply will be sufficient to meet the needs of the people. Such plans must aim to supply not only present requirements, but also those of the future — which are likely to be greater in most countries owing to population growth and increase in purchasing power.

The recommended intakes can also serve as a guide for drawing up ration scales for institutions, such as hospitals, orphanages, boarding schools, and prisons, as well as for the armed services. They may be useful as well in planning food for expeditions.

The figures for recommended intakes may be compared with actual consumption figures determined by food-consumption surveys. Such comparisons, though always useful, cannot in themselves justify statements that undernutrition, malnutrition, or overnutrition is present in a community or group, as such conclusions must always be supported by clinical or biochemical evidence. The recommended intakes are not an adequate yardstick for assessing health because — as will become apparent from the text — each figure represents an average requirement augmented by a factor that takes into account inter-individual variability. The recommended intakes are therefore the amounts considered sufficient for the maintenance of health in nearly all people.

FOOD WASTAGE

It must be understood that the recommendations apply to amounts of nutrients required by people in their stomachs. For many foodstuffs the journey from the fields where they are grown to the homes where they are eaten is a long one, and nutrient losses may occur on the farm, in barns and warehouses, in food factories, and in wholesale and retail distribution. Estimates of such losses can be made at a national level.

Food losses also inevitably occur in the home due to spoilage, methods of cooking and preparing meals, or plate waste. In homes with poor cooking equipment and storage facilities such losses are often unavoidable. The extent of these losses is hard to measure or estimate. Plate waste is certainly closely related to food availability. In a home where food is scarce and the family often hungry not more than one percent may be wasted in this way. On the other hand inspection of garbage cans outside some houses in affluent suburbs would suggest that such families acquire more food than their members consume. Ten percent is probably the representative figure for wastage in homes where reasonable care is taken.

SOME EFFECTS OF UNDERFEEDING AND OVERFEEDING

All mammals, including primitive man, developed in environments where the food supply was uncertain and temporary restrictions in food intake were a normal experience. Man has evolved with reserves and adaptive mechanisms which help him to survive periods of famine. His reserves of energy in the form of carbohydrate are small and may be exhausted by two days of starvation, but if he has been previously well fed, the reserves of fat supply sufficient energy to prevent death from starvation for two months or longer. By contrast, a man may die from cold in two or three hours or from lack of water in two or three days. These facts should help in fixing priorities when planning relief measures after a large natural disaster. For someone in good health two weeks with no food is a most unpleasant experience, but it has no permanent adverse effects on health, as participants in hunger strikes well know. If the period of food deprivation is prolonged, the need for energy is reduced by deliberate curtailment of all unnecessary physical activity; moreover, as starvation proceeds, the tissues waste and the body becomes smaller, thus needing less energy to maintain itself.

The body has no real store of protein; however, as a tissue wastes, the proteins in it are broken down and the constituent amino acids become available, at least in part, to maintain the protein in other and more essential tissues and cells. Furthermore, the cells, especially those of the liver, adapt so that the amino acids from a limited supply of protein can be utilized more readily for the function of maintenance and less as a source of energy. In a normal adult the protein losses from the body are not likely to become critical until the body weight has fallen by at least 25 percent, which usually does not occur before about two months of total starvation.

Most of the water-soluble vitamins are attached as cofactors or apoproteins. If the body lacks a supply of a vitamin from the outside, clinical signs of deficiency appear when a vital biochemical function has been impaired. Scurvy or beriberi or pellagra may be expected to appear after varying periods of time in a community suddenly cut off from a supply of ascorbic acid or thiamine or niacin, respectively. On the contrary, the liver of a healthy adult contains stores of vitamin B_{12} and vitamin A sufficient to last for many months or even years.

Only in recent years have some large communities had ample supplies of foods made easily available to them with little expenditure of physical energy. Furthermore, many foods have been made more than normally appetizing by artificial means. In such communities there is thus every possibility and temptation to eat more than is required. Since the body has no other means of disposing of excess energy in the food than by storing it as fat, obesity, with its adverse effect on health, is now widespread among children, adolescents, and adults in some countries.

Because excess dietary protein is readily converted into amino acids and subsequently used as energy, it does not accumulate in the body. The traditional diets of some communities — for example, the South American gauchos, the East African Masai tribe, and the Eskimos — consist almost entirely of meat and other foods of animal origin. These diets may provide 200 g of protein per day, more than double the normal intake, without causing any apparent harm. However, in new foods from unconventional sources, such as yeast and chlorella, a green alga which grows in the scum on ponds, the protein is associated with large amounts of nucleic acids. These break down to form uric acid, which may give rise to kidney stones if large quantities of such proteins are eaten.

Any dietary excess of the water-soluble vitamins is readily excreted in the urine; hence, poisoning from these vitamins is unknown. This method of disposal is not available to the fat-soluble vitamins, but very large amounts of vitamin A can be stored in the liver. Both vitamins A and D are, however, potentially detrimental, and the well-known effects of overdosage with medicinal preparations are to be discussed later in this text.

The minerals calcium and iron are required by the body in the manufacture of bone and haemoglobin, the pigment present in the red blood corpuscles. Both calcium and iron are present in the diet in much greater quantities than are needed by the body, whereas the kidneys can excrete into the urine only limited amounts of calcium and negligible amounts of iron. The body's requirements of these two minerals are met by means of two control mechanisms in the small intestine which regulate absorption, and the greater part of the dietary intake of both elements passes straight through the intestines and is lost in the faeces. The nature of neither of the two control mechanisms is well understood, but both normally work with precision. Certain diseases may cause them to break down, as a result of which insufficient calcium or iron is absorbed. Each mechanism has a large reserve capacity for rejecting an excess dietary intake, but under certain circumstances it may be inadequate.

It is very difficult to assess precisely the dietary needs for protein, vitamins, and minerals because individuals vary in their needs. For this reason, as has already been mentioned, the recommended intakes each include a safety factor. Any excess intake not required by the body is used in the case of protein as a source of energy, in the case of water-soluble vitamins excreted in the urine, in the case of vitamin A stored in the liver, and in the case of calcium and iron not absorbed in the small intestine but rejected in the faeces.

None of these considerations apply to energy intake in food. Each individual, so as to meet exactly his requirement, must be regulated by his appetite or his feeding habits. If his intake is for any reason below requirement, he becomes thin and wastes away; if his intake is above requirement, he becomes fat and is exposed to all the health hazards of obesity. Consequently there is no safety factor in recommendations for energy intake, although requirements may vary among individuals of the same sex and age.

2. ENERGY

The human body is an engine which can set free the chemical energy bound in fuels present in foods. These are carbohydrates, fats, proteins, and alcohol. Since the body continually converts and replaces its component parts, energy is needed for the synthesis of new organic substances in this continuing process of maintenance. The synthetic reactions which produce the chemical components of the new cells and tissues during growth also require energy, and the faster the rate of growth the greater the need for fuel. The body also has to have energy for internal work, such as the action of the heart in circulating the blood and the movements of the diaphragm in breathing. Less obvious is the work done in maintaining the concentrations of salts and ions in the cells and body fluids. Sodium and chloride are the main ions in the blood, and potassium and phosphate in the cells. The difference in the ionic composition of the fluids inside and outside the cells is essential to their normal functioning and can only be maintained by chemical reactions utilizing energy. All these processes constitute the resting energy exchanges, also known as *basal metabolism*, which is equal to the energy expenditure when the body is at complete rest.

Additional fuel is needed for external work performed by the muscles, such as moving the body about, maintaining its posture, lifting and carrying loads, and the varied physical activities of everyday life.

It has been customary to express the energy content of foods and the energy requirements of man and animals in terms of the thermochemical kilocalorie (this unit is usually referred to loosely as simply the "kilocalorie" or even the "calorie"). The thermochemical calorie was originally defined as the quantity of heat required to raise the temperature of 1 g of water from 14.5°C to 15.5°C, but it is now defined in terms of the joule: 1 cal_{th} = 4.184 O J. The thermochemical kilocalorie is 10^3 times this value — that is, 4.184 O kJ (kilojoules). Conversely, 1 kJ = 0.239 kcal and 1 MJ = 1 000 kJ = 239 kcal.

In the International System of Units (SI) the unit of work, energy, or quantity of heat is the joule, which is the work done by a force of one newton in displacing through a distance of one metre the point to which it is applied. Since the newton is the force that will impart to a mass of 1 kg an acceleration of $1 \text{ m} \cdot \text{s}^{-2}$, the joule may be defined in terms of SI base units as $1 \text{ J} = \text{N} \cdot \text{m} = 1 \text{ m}^2 \cdot \text{kg} \cdot \text{s}^{-2}$. Energy requirements are increasingly being given in joules. The energy content of diets and energy requirements of humans usually exceed 1 000 kJ and are generally expressed in terms of megajoules (MJ).

The approximate energy values of the body fuels are the following: for carbohydrate, 4 kcal or 16.7 kJ per gram; for fat, 9 kcal or 37.7 kJ per gram; for protein, 4 kcal or 16.7 kJ per gram; and for alcohol, 7 kcal or 29.3 kJ per gram. These are net values, allowing for the small losses of energy in the faeces and also for the energy lost in the urine in the form of urea and other nitrogenous end-products of protein metabolism which cannot be completely broken up in the body.

The energy content of a foodstuff is obtained by applying the above factors to its carbohydrate, fat, protein, and — where applicable — alcohol content as determined by chemical analysis. Tables of food analysis are available for many countries and regions of the world, and there are, in addition, international and regional food-composition tables prepared by FAO, of which those for Latin America, Africa, East Asia, and the Near East are examples. Compilers of such tables may use slightly different and more accurate figures than those given above, which are only approximations, the figures being rounded off so that they can be remembered easily; but their use is unlikely to involve any serious error.

The subject of the metabolism of alcohol in humans and laboratory animals has been investigated from time to time. The purpose of these studies has been to determine whether alcohol may serve the same purpose in the energy economy as ordinary carbohydrate does in saving protein and in providing energy for muscular activity, the deposition of fat, and the generation of heat to maintain body temperature.

It has been observed that under conditions of moderate intake most of the potential energy of the ingested alcohol is available for muscular work and for the production of body heat. The partial replacement of carbohydrate or fat in the diet by an amount of alcohol equal in energy content has also been shown to be effective in the synthesis of body tissue.

The body can oxidize alcohol at a limited rate. A healthy, well-fed adult who in terms of body weight consumes alcohol in quantities of less than 2 g/kg in twenty-four hours oxidizes it at a constant but limited rate of about 100 mg/kg per hour. A 65-kg man and a 55-kg woman can thus obtain, respectively, 700 kcal (2.9 MJ) and 525 kcal (2.2 MJ) daily from alcohol.

ENERGY REQUIREMENTS OF ADULTS

It is convenient to consider the expenditure and thereby the requirements of persons of different occupation, age, and size by reference to a man and woman 25 years of age and weighing 65 kg and 55 kg, respectively. Assuming that one spends eight hours each in bed, at work, and in nonoccupational activities, the total energy expenditures of our reference man and woman can be calculated. Tables 2 and 3 illustrate how their energy expenditures may be distributed over twenty-four hours and the effect of occupation.

While at rest in bed the energy expended approximates the basal metabolic rate (BMR) — for the reference man a little over 1 kcal/min, and for the reference woman a little under 1 kcal/min. This rate is increased by about one-half when sitting and using the arms for light work. It is doubled when standing and moving about slowly, and quadrupled when walking at a brisk pace. Thus the rate of energy expenditure when one is on foot and carrying out domestic and everyday tasks is between two and four times the resting rate. Similar rates of work are found in light industry. With heavy work, such as using a pick and shovel or moving big loads, the rate may rise to eight times the resting level. Exceptionally heavy work in industry and first-rate performance in some sports may raise energy expenditure to sixteen times or occasionally twenty times the resting level, but such rates are possible only for specially trained persons and, then, only for short periods.

The energy expended during the eight hours at work is thus determined by occupation and affected only to a small degree by the individual. A rough classification of the different occupations by level of activity is given on the following page.

KG. — 2. 2046 pds.   man = 143 pds.
woman = 122 pds.

Light

Men: Office workers, most professionals (lawyers, doctors, accountants, teachers, architects, etc.), shop workers, the unemployed.

Women: Office workers, housewives with mechanical household appliances, teachers and most other professionals.

Moderately active

Men: Most men in light industry, students, construction workers (excluding heavy labourers), many farm workers, soldiers not on active service, fishermen.

Women: Workers in light industry, housewives without mechanical household appliances, students, department-store workers.

Very active

Men: Some agricultural workers, unskilled labourers, forestry workers, army recruits, soldiers on active service, mine workers, steel workers, athletes.

Women: Some farm workers (especially in peasant agriculture), dancers, athletes.

Exceptionally active

Men: Lumberjacks, blacksmiths, rickshaw pullers.
Women: Construction workers.

The energy expenditure per hour by men and women for light work is 140 and 100 kcal (0.58 and 0.41 MJ), respectively; for moderately active work, 175 and 125 kcal (0.73 and 0.51 MJ); for very active work, 240 and 175 kcal (1.0 and 0.74 MJ); and for exceptionally active work, 300 and 225 kcal (1.25 and 0.94 MJ).

The expenditure of energy during the recreational or nonoccupational period is determined in large part by individual choice. It can range anywhere between 700 and 1 500 kcal (3.0 and 6.3 MJ) for men and 580 and 980 kcal (2.4 and 4.1 MJ) for women for an eight-hour period, depending on the type of activity. In an industrial society an individual's energy requirements are determined more by his choice of recreation than by his occupation. Assuming that our reference man and woman engage in some moderately active recreations, their daily energy expenditure works out to 3 000 kcal (12.5 MJ) and 2 200 kcal (9.2 MJ), respectively.

In addition to physical activity and to the type and nature of non-occupational activities, the energy requirements of individuals depend as well on the following variables, which are interrelated in a complex way: (a) body size and composition; (b) age; and (c) climate and other ecological factors.

Body size and composition

Energy expenditure may be influenced by the effect of body size and composition on (a) resting metabolism, (b) the physical effort of moving the whole body or large parts of the body, and (c) the work of standing, of maintaining posture, and of small movements of the limbs. Also, the total physical activity of an individual may be influenced by the quantity of adipose tissue in his body. When the body composition is normal, the energy requirement of adults per unit of body weight is the same: for moderately active men 46 kcal (0.19 MJ) per kilogram of body weight, and for moderately active women 40 kcal (0.17 MJ) per kilogram of body weight. The energy requirement of very active and exceptionally active men and women per unit of body weight is much higher. Because women have a larger proportion of fat, their energy requirement is less than that of men.

Age

The energy expenditure of adults may alter with age because of (a) changes in body weight or body composition, (b) a decrease in the basal metabolic rate, (c) a decline in physical activity, and (d) an increasing prevalence of disease and disabilities. In many populations the amount of body fat and the total body weight tend to increase with age; this may affect the basal metabolism and, hence, the total energy requirements.

There is little evidence that physical activity, either at work or at leisure, alters significantly between the ages of 20 and 39. From the age of 40 onward several changes may occur. Older people tend to leave work that requires high energy expenditure or to be less active in such occupations. Even in occupations with moderate requirements, physical activity at work may be slightly reduced. Physical activity during the nonoccupational period of the day is likely to diminish with advancing age, and most people further reduce their physical activity after the age of 60. For people 60 to 69 years of age the limitation of physical activity attributable to disease or disability is highly variable, and it becomes even more so after the age of 70.

The FAO/WHO Expert Committee on Energy and Protein Requirements recommended that the average energy requirement of men and women be regarded as unchanging from 20 to 39 years of age. The energy requirement decreases by 5 percent for each decade between the ages of 40 and 59 and by 10 percent from 60 to 69 years of age; for age 70 and above another reduction of 10 percent is suggested.

Climate

That human beings eat less food in a hot climate than they do in a cold climate is generally recognized, but it is extremely difficult to express the relationship between climate and food needs quantitatively. First of all, there is no good method of assessing the overall climatic stress; secondly, the degree of protection against the climate varies greatly. In industrial societies in cold climates, where homes, factories, offices, cars, and trains are artificially heated, many people are exposed to the cold for only a few minutes daily, and even then they are fully protected by good clothing. In hot climates the air conditioning of homes, offices, and factories is on the increase, but still benefits only a minority of the population.

The FAO/WHO Expert Committee on Protein and Energy Requirements considered that there was no quantifiable basis for correcting rest and exercise requirements according to climate. When physical activity is restricted by environmental factors, the category of activity should be adjusted accordingly.

ENERGY REQUIREMENTS OF INFANTS, CHILDREN, AND ADOLESCENTS

Infants

As human milk of good quality and in sufficient quantity is the normal food of the full-term infant, he is more likely to thrive smoothly on it than on any other food. The energy requirements of infants during the first six months of life can be estimated from the observed intakes of breast-fed infants who are growing normally. It is recognized that there is a notable day-to-day variation in energy intake, both between babies and for the same baby, caused by variations in the volume and energy content of milk. The individual requirement also varies largely depending on the activeness of the child. The mean energy requirements of an infant during the first year are as follows:

Age	kcal/kg	kJ/kg
< 3 months	120	500
3-5 "	115	480
6-8 "	110	460
9-11 "	105	440
Mean for first year	112	470

Children and adolescents

The energy expenditure of children is difficult to measure accurately because of their varied and ever changing range of physical activities. The energy intake of children must obviously allow for satisfactory growth and physical development and for the high degree of activity that is characteristic of healthy children. Recommendations for the energy requirements of children are based mainly on measurements of the actual food intakes of healthy children who are growing normally.

During adolescence both girls and boys grow at a faster rate than at any other time except infancy. The calorie requirements of a boy during the time he is approaching manhood are higher than at any other time in his life. Those of a girl approaching womanhood are exceeded only during pregnancy and lactation. During this period of adolescence — the manifestations of which may be much more striking in an individual child than average figures indicate — there is an increase in the apparent basal metabolic requirement, which includes the growth requirement. This increased caloric need is ordinarily reflected in the appetite.

A practical problem arises in connection with the requirements of a community where a significant proportion of the children are underweight because of previous malnutrition. Since the intention is to provide for catch-up growth, a return to the normal height and weight, it might be reasoned that allowances should be calculated on the basis of age rather than weight. This reasoning does apply up to the age of puberty; but older children who have been malnourished are unlikely ever to catch up and reach normal size, and the consumption of extra food would only lead to obesity. It is therefore suggested that after the thirteenth birthday the recommended intakes should be corrected only for actual body weight.

ENERGY REQUIREMENTS DURING PREGNANCY AND LACTATION

During pregnancy extra energy is needed for the growth of the foetus, as well as the placenta and associated maternal tissues, and for the increased cost of movement for the heavier mother. Basal metabolism rises by 20 percent in the last trimester of pregnancy. The total energy cost to meet the increased needs of pregnancy is about 80 000 kcal (335 MJ), which means an average increase of 285 kcal (1.2 MJ) per day over the 280 days of pregnancy, or about 150 kcal (0.6 MJ) per day in the first trimester and 350 kcal (1.5 MJ) per day during the second and third trimesters.

For many women the burden of pregnancy is added to the physical work of running a home and caring for several small children, and in such cases additional food is needed to meet all the energy requirements of pregnancy. On the other hand, there are women with little or no household work who give up a job or active recreation and lead a sedentary life when they become pregnant. In these circumstances a pregnant woman may actually need less food than before. For many women some curtailment of activity occurs, so the total 80 000 kcal (335 MJ) of extra energy may not be needed.

The mean daily milk production is about 850 ml, having an energy value of roughly 600 kcal (2.5 MJ). If the efficiency of milk production is about 80 percent, a mother will need 750 kcal (3.1 MJ) from food to meet the needs of lactation. Since a reserve energy of 36 000 kcal (151 MJ), deposited as fat during pregnancy is available for lactation, the additional energy requirement for lactation will be 550 kcal (2.3 MJ) per day. For twin pregnancy and simultaneous breast-feeding of more than one infant, additional requirements must be taken into account.

The recommended intakes of energy during the last half of pregnancy and the six months of lactation are given in Table 1.

Although a number of essential nutrients, such as proteins, vitamins, and minerals, should be considered in the selection of an adequate diet, it must not be forgotten that energy is fundamentally one of the most important as Du Bois pointed out:

Calories (energy) in medical practice are just as important as they ever were in spite of the fact that attention has been centered on vitamins. No supplements of vitamins or mineral elements can alter the laws of the conservation of energy. Calories (energy) are still needed to keep the body warm and to furnish energy for muscular work.

When emergencies arise, energy must be provided first in order to keep people alive and satisfied.

3. PROTEINS

Proteins are indispensable constituents of living protoplasm and as such participate in all vital processes. No living matter is devoid of protein. After water, protein is the major component of body tissue.

Proteins are large molecules made up of nitrogen-containing amino acids that are united together by peptide linkage. It was first assumed that all forms of proteins were similar in composition. This thinking continued until, in 1901, Emil Fisher showed that proteins are composed of amino acids that differ in arrangement and in qualitative relationships.

Of the 22 amino acids now known to be physiologically important, the body is capable of synthesizing some under proper conditions and if a supply of nitrogen is made available. These amino acids are known as the dispensable, or nonessential, amino acids. Others cannot be synthesized by the body and must therefore be supplied by diet. These are the indispensable, or essential, amino acids — leucine, isoleucine, lysine, methionine, phenylalanine, threonine, tryptophan, and valine. To these may be added histidine, which appears to be essential to the growth of infants.

MAJOR FUNCTIONS

1. Proteins are essential to growth. Fats and carbohydrates cannot be substituted for protein as they do not contain nitrogen.
2. Proteins provide the essential amino acids, which are the building stones for tissue synthesis. The body is constantly undergoing wear and tear which is repaired by proteins.
3. Proteins supply raw materials for the formation of digestive juices, hormones, plasma proteins, haemoglobin, vitamins, and enzymes.
4. Proteins can be used for energy purposes. Each gram of protein supplies about 4 kcal (16.7 kJ) of energy. It is, however, wasteful of protein to use it for such purposes.

5. Proteins function as buffers, thus helping to maintain the reactions of various media, such as plasma, cerebrospinal fluid, and intestinal secretions.

CLASSIFICATION OF PROTEINS

Proteins can be classified as either *animal proteins* or *vegetable proteins*. Animal proteins contain more of the essential amino acids than vegetable proteins and, in general, have a higher nutritive value. More recent knowledge of the biological differences among amino acids has led to the classification of proteins as *biologically complete* or as *biologically incomplete*. A biologically complete protein is one which contains all of the essential amino acids in adequate amounts to meet human requirements. A biologically incomplete protein is deficient in one or more of the essential amino acids. This deficiency may be either absolute or relative. Most of the vegetable proteins lack one or more of the essential amino acids and are thus classified as biologically incomplete proteins, although mixtures of vegetable proteins may present all of the amino acids in adequate quantities. Therefore, the various proteins may complement one another as long as they are not all lacking in the same amino acid.

After ingestion, dietary proteins are acted upon by proteolytic enzymes (pepsin, trypsin, and chymotrypsin) and converted into amino acids, which are absorbed and used for tissue synthesis or the formation of enzymes, certain hormones, and other proteins of special significance. The ultimate fate of the amino acids is the removal of nitrogen for the formation of urea and their direct or indirect release as energy.

PROTEIN REQUIREMENTS

The subject of protein requirements had been discussed at a number of national and international conferences — most recently in 1971 by the Joint FAO/WHO Expert Group on Energy and Protein Requirements.

Adult requirements

Since there is a cessation of growth in adults, they require protein only for maintenance purposes. The body of an adult contains

18-19 percent protein. The proteins are continuously broken down and replaced in the tissues, but this process occurs at very different rates in the various organs. For example, the epithelial lining of the intestinal tract is renewed every three or four days, whereas collagen — the protein present in tendons, bones, and connective tissues — is turned over very slowly, with individual molecules possibly remaining unchanged for many years. The total turnover of proteins in a human adult amounts to about 400 g per day. The proteins released in this turnover are broken down into their constituent amino acids, most of which can be used again in the manufacture of new protein molecules; however, a fraction is further broken down, and the nitrogen present is converted into urea and other products which are lost in the urine. The total obligatory loss of nitrogen (N) from the body due to the above and other losses amounts to 2 mg N/kcal or 0.48 mg N/kJ of basal metabolism. The protein requirements of an adult can be experimentally determined from the losses of nitrogen when the subjects are fed a nitrogen-free diet.

The Joint FAO/WHO Expert Group which met in 1971 carefully studied the data obtained with this "factorial approach," as well as from nitrogen-balance studies, and arrived at a figure of 0.57 g and 0.52 g per day for each kilogram of body weight as the safe level of protein intake in terms of cow's milk or egg protein for an adult man or woman. The safe level of intake is the amount shown to have been necessary to meet the physiological needs and maintain the health of nearly all individuals in the group and is therefore higher than the average protein requirements.

Moreover, populations do subsist mainly on mixed proteins of vegetable and animal origin, rather than on the egg or milk proteins used to express the safe levels of protein intake. The nutritive value of such mixed dietary proteins, which is generally lower than that of milk or egg proteins, can be determined by biological methods. When using safe levels of protein intake to assess needs in terms of dietary protein, correction for protein quality is necessary, as in the following formula:

$$\text{Requirement of dietary protein} = \frac{\text{safe level of protein intake} \times \text{protein value of egg}}{\text{protein value of dietary protein}}$$

Since vegetable proteins possess a lower nutritive value, more such protein is required to satisfy the requirements.

Man derives protein not from a single source but from a variety of sources. It is now well recognized that proteins from different sources mutually supplement each other, as a result of which blends of two or more proteins may possess a higher biological value than the individual proteins. A strong warning should be sounded against the condemnation of a food because, when eaten alone, its proteins do not have a high biological value.

The diets of low-income groups are based mainly on cereals. The proteins of cereals are often low in biological value owing to the fact that most of them have a low content of one or more essential amino acids — for example, maize is low in tryptophan and lysine, rice in lysine and threonine, and wheat in lysine. In most parts of the world cereal-based diets traditionally include small amounts of legumes. Legumes contain as much as 25 percent protein that is rich in lysine, thus supplementing the lysine-deficient cereal proteins. Diets based on a mixture of cereals and legumes therefore possess a protein nutritive value that is significantly higher than those based on cereals or legumes alone.

As a community prospers, its diet becomes more and more varied and the consumption of cereals falls. Higher consumption of animal protein foods — like meat, milk, eggs, and fish — and of fats and oils increases the energy level of the diet and thus furthers protein utilization. Animal proteins, in addition to being complete and more nutritive, have a significant supplementary value in relation to vegetable proteins, most of which are deficient in the essential amino acid lysine. Thus animal proteins could be used to effectively supplement poor diets based on foods of vegetable origin. It must be pointed out here that practical nutrition is concerned with the nutritive value of diets, not of individual foods.

The value of the proteins in meat and milk as supplements to grain products is illustrated by a study with rats. Equal parts of animal protein from meat or milk and vegetable protein from white whole-wheat or rye flour are seen to give as good growth as meat or milk alone. The supplementary value of whole milk, skim-milk solids, and cheese proteins to bread and potatoes has also been effectively demonstrated by biological studies with experimental animals. The protein requirement for humans can no doubt be met most effectively by mixtures of plant and animal proteins. Well-balanced mixtures of plant proteins may also maintain individuals in good health over a long period of time. It should be recognized, however, that persons consuming diets based mainly on animal protein foods or a mixture of animal and vegetable protein foods require lesser amounts of dietary protein for maintenance as compared to those whose diets are based solely on vegetable protein foods.

The safe levels of protein intake in terms of milk or egg protein for maintenance of an adult man and woman are 0.57 g and 0.52 g per kilogram of body weight per day. This works out to 37 g per day for a reference man weighing 65 kg and 29 g per day for a reference woman weighing 55 kg. All estimates of protein requirements are valid only when energy requirements are fully met. If the total energy intake is inadequate, some dietary protein is used for energy and is therefore not available to satisfy protein needs. Further increasing protein intakes to meet safe levels is of limited effectiveness and wasteful if energy needs are not being satisfied at the same time.

For persons engaging in heavy manual work the energy needs are higher. Consequently, the total food intake is greater, and normally there is an increased intake of protein. Yet, there is no satisfactory evidence of an increased protein need resulting from greater physical activity per se. Athletes in training and others who augment their physical activity are also increasing their muscle mass and so need some additional protein during this period; however, the additional amount of protein needed is not likely to be large.

Infections and infestations affect protein requirements by inducing some depletion of body nitrogen. The quantitative effects of acute episodes of infectious diseases on the protein needs of an individual cannot be stated, as they are likely to vary with frequency, severity, and nature of the infection and with other host factors, including nutritional status.

Growth requirements

Protein requirements during infancy, childhood, and adolescence are greater than those of adults owing to the necessity of maintaining healthy growth rates. The weight of an infant doubles during the first six months of life and trebles during the first twelve months, after which the growth rate declines considerably until adolescence. The weight gained per kilogram of body weight is 5-6 g per day in the first six months of life, falling to about 2-3 g in the second six months of life, 0.5-0.6 g in the second year, and 0.3 g in the sixth year, thereafter remaining at about this figure until adolescence.

When breast-fed by a healthy well-nourished mother with normal lactation, the newborn child consumes adequate amounts and quality of dietary protein to meet his protein requirements. The efficiency of utilization of mother's milk by the infant is assumed to be 100 percent.

The daily protein requirements per kilogram of body weight of a child during the first year of life are as follows:

Months	Grams *
< 3	2.40
3-6	1.85
6-9	1.62
9-11	1.44

* In terms of milk or egg protein.

If proteins of lower quality than those of milk are fed, the intakes should be proportionately higher, although obviously every effort should be made to provide the infant with the highest possible quality of protein.

In the next four years, up to the fifth birthday, the child gradually comes to eat the normal food of the family, but milk should remain an important part of his diet during this period. After the age of five, when the growth rate slows down, a child thrives on a normal adult diet, provided it is ample and the protein mixture is of good quality.

Allowances for pregnancy and lactation

It is widely recognized that the nutrition of the pregnant woman has an important influence on the course of the pregnancy and the health of the infant. The average birth weight is relatively low in many poor countries, while birth weights in the upper socio-economic groups of these countries are similar to the average birth weights that are characteristic of rich countries. Low birth weights are thus related to conditions of poverty, including poor nutrient intakes during pregnancy. An additional daily allowance of 6 g of good-quality protein, such as that of milk or egg, would cover the extra needs of all women during pregnancy.

The additional protein needed by the lactating woman can be estimated from the volume and composition of the milk secreted. There is no evidence that the synthesis of milk protein is either more or less efficient than the synthesis of other body proteins. During the first six months of full lactation the average volume of milk secreted is 850 ml per day. As human milk contains an average of 1.2 g of protein per 100 ml, the protein content of the daily secretion is about 10 g. An additional allowance of 17 g of protein of the same quality as that of milk or egg covers the extra needs of lactation.

MEETING PROTEIN NEEDS

When man's food consumption is not restricted by the availability of foodstuffs or by economic circumstances, he tends to choose a diet that provides about 11 percent of its energy value from proteins. This should be remembered in practical planning, since a level of dietary protein of this general magnitude based upon a protein mixture including proteins of animal origin, might both meet protein requirements and completely satisfy human desires as regards the composition of the diet. This is the most practical advice that can be offered at this time.

The diet of growing children and of pregnant and lactating mothers should contain adequate amounts of milk to meet their protein demands. The value of milk in providing good nutrition to the vulnerable groups of the population is well known. A great problem of our times is that in many countries the human population has outgrown the population of dairy cattle.

The building up of dairy herds takes many years. In large areas of the world it is impractical to conceive of supplies of dairy milk meeting population needs in the near future. Alternatives became available with the discovery of the possibility of making milk substitutes from mixtures of vegetable proteins (soya, peanut, etc.). Many of these preparations are suitable for supplemental feeding of children.

Also, there are now available protein foods based on blends of cereal flours, oil-seed meals, legume flours, and skim-milk powder, adequately fortified with vitamins and minerals, which can be used as effective supplements to the diets of preschool children and pregnant and lactating mothers.

In many of the developing countries the lack of sufficient quantities of nutritious foods, coupled with the prevalence of infections and other diseases, has led to a high incidence of protein-calorie malnutrition. The majority of children in the developing countries grow very satisfactorily up to six months of age, and their weight and general development is comparable with that of children of the developed countries. This satisfactory situation exists because the protein and other nutrient requirements of these infants are met from breast milk. After the age of six months the infant's overall need for protein increases due to the demands of growth and the development of muscular tissue. If the increased protein requirements are not met during this period, the infant will experience a growth failure. Furthermore, if the protein deficiency of the diet is acute, symptoms of protein-calorie malnutrition will set in. Recent researches indicate that under such stress conditions it is not only physical development that suffers, but learning capacity as well.

PLANNING FOR NATIONAL PROTEIN NEEDS

When predicting food demands at a national level, it must be borne in mind that because humans seem to have a desire for proteins, individual intakes are often considerably above the suggested safe levels. Such demands on the part of the wealthier sectors of a community may well influence the economic availability of protein and hence the distribution of intake among population groups.

The national protein needs in terms of egg or milk protein can easily be calculated on the basis of the distribution and respective requirements of the population by age groups. These calculations have certain limitations, however. In practice, concern about protein intake is for the most part directed to the younger age groups in the population. Examination of national protein supplies tells relatively little about the supply of protein to specific population groups. Planning should be based upon an examination of the nutrient intake of the population, particularly that of vulnerable groups, and this information should be incorporated into the planning process for economic and social development.

4. VITAMINS

Vitamins are organic substances which the body requires in small amounts and yet cannot make for itself; hence, they have to be provided by the diet.

The term vitamin was introduced in 1912 by the Polish biochemist Casimir Funk with the belief that all these substances were "vital amines"; however, it was soon shown that most of the vitamins are unrelated chemically and that only a few of them are amines. At first, as the vitamins were discovered, they were identified by letters of the alphabet. Later, as each vitamin was isolated in pure form and its chemical structure was determined, it was given a chemical name. These chemical names are now their correct designations, although the original and more familiar letters are still used as in the following examples:

vitamin A_1	retinol
vitamin B_1	thiamine
vitamin B_2	riboflavine
vitamin B_{12}	cyanocobalamin
vitamin C	ascorbic acid
vitamin D_3	cholecalciferol

The nomenclature of the B group of vitamins has a complicated history. The pioneers in its study discovered that a watery extract of yeast given to rats on artificial diets containing no natural foods promoted growth. Such diets were said to contain vitamin B. The extracts were soon divided into two components: vitamin B_1, readily destroyed by heat, which was seen to prevent the appearance of disturbances of the nervous system in rats fed on the artificial diets and also became known as the antineuritic or antiberiberi vitamin; and vitamin B_2, resistant to heat, which was seen to prevent the appearance of dermatitis in rats. Vitamin B_2 was subsequently subdivided into two factors. One of these, riboflavine, is still sometimes called vitamin B_2. The other is known as the PP factor, because it prevents pellagra from appearing in man. Nicotinic acid, or niacin, was later shown to possess PP activity; it is usually found in foods in the form of its amide, nicotinamide, which is also active against pellagra.

As a result of further studies, up to twelve B vitamins have been postulated at one time or another. Many of these have failed to survive detailed investigation, but thiamine, riboflavine, niacin, pyridoxine (vitamin B_6), folic acid (folate), and cyanocobalamin (vitamin B_{12}) are now firmly established, and all of them except pyridoxine are to be discussed in this chapter. Pyridoxine is made up of a group of derivatives of pyridine, so widely distributed in foods that it is extremely rare for a human being to show signs of deficiency; however, convulsions have been observed in certain infants to be due to a deficiency of pyridoxine. The National Research Council in the U.S.A. has recommended an allowance of 2 mg per day of pyridoxine for an adult, which provides a good margin of safety. No recommendation has yet been made by FAO/WHO.

There are other natural substances related to retinol and cholecalciferol which have vitamin A and vitamin D activity. Vitamins A_1, A_2, D_2, and D_3 have been chemically characterized. Beta carotene, present in dark leafy vegetables, is a precursor of vitamin A and possesses significant vitamin A activity. In nearly all human diets almost all vitamin A and D activity is provided by retinol and beta carotene and by cholecalciferol, respectively.

The FAO/WHO Expert Groups have considered human requirements for eight vitamins: retinol, thiamine, niacin, riboflavine, cyanocobalamin, folate, ascorbic acid, and cholecalciferol. It is well known that diets lacking in each of these vitamins are consumed by man in readily definable circumstances. Furthermore, the effect on health of a lack of each of these vitamins can be recognized clinically. At least as many other vitamins which are necessary to man have not been considered by an FAO/WHO Expert Group and are therefore not discussed in this manual. At present, naturally occurring deficiency diseases have not been identified for these other vitamins, and it has been assumed that usual diets supply adequate or near-adequate amounts of these nutrients. Clinical deficiencies of some — for example, vitamin B_6 (pyridoxine) — are known, but these have been seen under highly unusual conditions or as secondary to another disease or to an inborn error of metabolism. Thus major attention has been focused upon the vitamins discussed in this handbook, all of which are involved in deficiency diseases observed in the general population.

Vitamins have long been classified into two groups: *water-soluble* and *fat-soluble*. This division is still useful, since it helps us understand the distribution of the vitamins in foods. There is also an important distinction in the handling of the two classes by the body. Any excess intake of the water-soluble vitamins is readily dissolved by the kidneys and excreted in the urine. Thus there is virtually no danger in being given an excess of these vitamins. On the other hand, the fat-soluble vitamins cannot be excreted in this way. Any excess beyond the immediate requirements is stored in solution in the fat in the liver. The storage capacity of the human liver is large, and it normally holds a reserve of vitamin A sufficient for many months; this is a useful provision against times when the dietary supply may temporarily be cut off. The amount that can be stored is not unlimited, however.

Concentrated preparations of vitamins A and D are easily obtainable. Mothers who are overanxious for the nutritional well-being of their children may poison them with excessive doses of these preparations.

Retinol (vitamin A₁)

Vitamin A — which occurs in two forms, designated A_1 and A_2 — has several functions in the body. One which is well understood concerns the pigment rhodopsin, or visual purple, present in the retina, or internal lining, of the eye. Retinol (vitamin A_1) is an alcohol, and the aldehyde derived from it is an essential part of visual purple. This pigment is bleached by light, a process which stimulates the rods in the retina, thereby enabling a person to see in dim light. Vitamin A deficiency leads to night blindness; this in itself is not a serious condition, but it is a warning that more dangerous consequences of this vitamin deficiency, even total blindness, may follow. Night blindness is common in many parts of Southeast Asia, the Middle East, and tropical Africa.

Vitamin A is also essential for the maintenance of the epithelial cells which line the surfaces and cavities of the body. Deficiency of the vitamin causes these cells to flatten and heap up on one another and their surface to become dry. This condition is most readily visible on the conjunctiva, or outer lining of the eye, where it leads to a form of conjunctivitis known as *xerophthalmia* — a common disturbance, which, fortunately, is usually confined to the conjunctiva over the sclera, or white of the eyeball. If it spreads to the cornea, vision is affected and the cornea may soften — a condition known as *keratomalacia*. If this process is not halted at once, the cornea perforates, the iris and also the lens may protrude through the gap, and permanent blindness follows almost invariably. Keratomalacia may occur at any age, but is usually found in children as a complication of severe forms of protein-calorie malnutrition. It has been estimated that twenty thousand children are permanently blinded in this way every year. Each of these tragedies could have been prevented by a little knowledge and timely care. Vitamin A deficiency may also result in *phrynoderma* or *follicular hyperkeratosis*, a condition characterized by common types of skin eruptions.

DIETARY SOURCES OF RETINOL

Retinol (vitamin A_1) is found only in foods of animal origin, but it can also be manufactured in the body from the pigments known as carotenes which are distributed widely in plants. One of these, beta carotene, is by far the most important source of retinol.

Since this vitamin is concentrated and stored in the liver fat, liver is a rich source, but meat and carcass fat contain only traces and are of little nutritional value in this regard. Fish livers are especially rich in retinol, and cod-liver oil is a traditional form of supplying this vitamin to children; halibut- and shark-liver oils are usually even richer sources. Milk is a fairly rich source of vitamin A_1, which is present as well in butter and cheese. Eggs also contain significant amounts.

Carotene is supplied by fruits and vegetables. Carrots and many dark-green vegetables are very good sources, although cabbage and lettuce contain little. In general, the more coloured a fruit the richer its carotene content.

Most cereals contain insignificant amounts of carotene, although the yellow varieties of maize contain small quantities. Vegetable oils are not a source of carotene, with the exceptions of corn oil, which may contain a little, and red-palm oil, which is very rich in it. The introduction of red palm trees (*Elaeis guineensis Jacq*) into areas where sources of carotene or retinol are otherwise scarce has proved a valuable means of preventing vitamin A deficiency.

In many countries margarine and other butter substitutes must by law be fortified with retinol and/or beta carotene, of which they are consequently as good a source as the best butter. The amount of retinol in butter varies, depending on the amount of carotene in the pasture on which the cow or other animal providing the milk has grazed.

RETINOL EQUIVALENTS

If injected into the body, 2 µg of beta carotene are equivalent to 1 µg of retinol. The absorption of dietary carotene from the intestines is highly uncertain, and in most circumstances probably no more than one third becomes available to the body. Hence, 6 µg of dietary beta carotene may be taken as a dietary equivalent of 1 µg of retinol. This is only a biological approximation, however, and in reporting the vitamin A activity of a diet, it is therefore best to give the carotene and retinol content separately. The total activity may then be expressed in retinol equivalents — that is, the total retinol content of the diet plus one sixth of the beta carotene content.

International units

Before the chemical nature of vitamin A was known, it was necessary to express vitamin A activity in arbitrary biological units. One international unit (i.u.) of vitamin A is equivalent to 0.3 µg of crystalline vitamin A alcohol, or retinol.

DIETARY REQUIREMENTS OF RETINOL EQUIVALENTS

The recommended intake is 300 µg of retinol equivalents per day for infants, rising to 750 µg for adults (Table 1). These figures are based on the amounts necessary to maintain or restore normal levels of retinol in the blood of subjects who have been on experimental diets containing no retinol or carotene. They are also formulated on the basis of observations of the incidence of night blindness and the retinol levels in the blood of people living in areas with highly diverse dietary supplies of the vitamin.

To obtain 750 μg of retinol equivalents, it would be necessary to drink some 250 ml of milk and eat about 30 g of butter, 50 g of dark-green leafy vegetables, 100 g of other vegetables, and 100 g of fruit. These amounts constitute the basis of a good diet, such as most of us like to eat, but it is obvious from the figures that many poor people in all countries do not receive the recommended intake. The recommendation is indeed a liberal one, but translated into terms of food supply and agricultural production, it provides a sensible target for agriculture.

As already indicated, vitamin A deficiency falls most heavily on the young child. Most children will have started their lives with an adequate store of retinol in their liver which they received from their mothers before birth, as retinol passes readily across the placenta. This store is increased by a good supply of breast milk or other milk. In all countries, but especially in those where the retinol supply is below the recommended intake, it is important to pay close attention to the diets of pregnant women and nursing mothers. If, as may be very likely, this does not reach the recommended intake (see Table 1), the additional amount needed should be provided without hesitation in the form of a supplement of a fish-liver oil or other concentrates. Similar supplements should be given to infants and young children.

One of the worst scandals of our time is that some twenty thousand young children go permanently blind every year because of the lack of minute amounts of retinol in their diets. In the world there is an abundance of retinol present in the liver of fishes. Collecting and processing it into a palatable form sufficient to meet the recommended intakes of all the children in the world would be a trivial and cheap technical achievement in comparison to sending a man to the moon. A much more difficult task is that of distributing it to the children in need and of educating their mothers to its value.

Cholecalciferol (vitamin D₃)

RICKETS AND VITAMIN D DEFICIENCY

Vitamin D — a group of several related vitamins — promotes the absorption of calcium from the small intestine and also plays an essential part in the mechanism for mineralizing bone. If an infant lacks the vitamin, his bones do not harden normally, especially at the growing ends. If the deficiency persists as the child gets bigger, the bones cannot bear the weight of the body, so bowlegs together with other deformities of the chest, spine, and pelvis develop. This disease is known as rickets.

Rickets has a long history, but thanks to preventive measures it is no longer a major cause of ill health in the world. The disease was first properly described in London about three hundred years ago, and it subsequently grew in importance. By the end of the nineteenth century a great number of children in the large industrial cities of northern and central Europe and North America were affected by it. Rickets was also prevalent in the larger Muslim cities, such as Cairo and Lahore, where women and children lived in purdah. Although cases could be found among children brought up in country villages, the disease was much less common and less severe than in the cities. A particularly important feature of rickets, even an apparently minor case where no deformity is apparent to the eye, is that the outlet to the pelvis may be so narrowed as to make childbirth difficult in subsequent years. The long, hard labour so commonly experienced by women fifty to a hundred years ago, which so often ended in death for both baby and mother, was often due to a pelvis narrowed by rickets.

In the industrialized countries the incidence of rickets began to decline early in the twentieth century, although a few mild cases are still seen occasionally in most large cities. In a few parts of the world, however, rickets is still considered a major problem in child health. The disease has been reported as not uncommon in many parts of Asia and Africa. It is difficult to interpret some of these reports because the criteria for diagnosing mild cases are not well established. But the presence of even a few mild cases in a community serves as a warning against relaxation of the preventive measures discussed in the following pages.

COD-LIVER OIL AND OTHER SOURCES OF THE VITAMIN

Cod-liver oil is a very old household remedy, which in the second half of the nineteenth century came into increasingly widespread use for " dosing " children. It was known to be good for rickets, but it was not until 1918 that Mellanby, in experiments on puppies, proved that rickets was a deficiency disease, which could be prevented by giving cod-liver oil, and that a vitamin was present in the oil.

Cod-liver oil is a good source of the vitamin. The standardized British pharmacopoeial oil contains 200 μg/100 ml (a useful figure to remember for reasons which are to be discussed later). Halibut and swordfish oil are even richer, and all fish-liver oils contain useful amounts. Among other animal foods, only liver, eggs, and butter contain useful amounts, while there are only traces in both human and cow's milk. Foods of plant origin do not contain this vitamin.

SUNLIGHT AND THE MANUFACTURE OF CHOLECALCIFEROL

The alternative and for most of us the more important supply of the vitamin is that manufactured in the skin. Cholecalciferol can be formed in the skin if it is exposed to the ultraviolet rays of the sun.

Rickets persists today for two reasons. In northern cities the amount of sunlight, especially during the long dark winters, is just barely adequate. In sunny parts of the world, it is often customary to keep infants and young children swaddled or indoors, which means they are not sufficiently exposed to the ultraviolet rays. While in theory a dietary supply of vitamin D appears to be unessential, in practice it is wise in countries far away from the equator to try to make sure that all infants and young children receive some vitamin from the diet. This also is true for communities where custom and habit prevent the exposure of children to sunlight.

RECOMMENDED INTAKES OF CHOLECALCIFEROL

A daily intake of 10 μg of cholecalciferol is recommended for infants and children up to their seventh birthday. This amount is certainly enough both to prevent rickets and to ensure that the dietary calcium is absorbed in sufficient amounts.

It would be extremely difficult to give a child a natural diet containing this amount, as he would soon tire of eggs, herring, and pilchards. It is possible, however, to increase the intake artificially in two ways. First, foods such as dried milk, liquid milk, infant cereal products, and margarine may be enriched with cholecalciferol. Such enrichment of food is common practice in some countries, but it is only possible where there is a well-developed food technology, and if adequate care is not taken, it may be dangerous. It has already been pointed out that cholecalciferol can be toxic. In 1952, in England, cases in which infants, usually between five and eight months old, lost their appetite and became wasted were observed. The level of calcium in the blood was raised, the kidneys and heart sometimes became calcified, and mental retardation was common. Many of these infants died. There is little doubt that overdosage of vitamin D was in most instances responsible for this condition, which is known as *hypercalcaemia*. Some of these infants and children appeared to be abnormally sensitive to vitamin D. When, a few years later, the U.K. Government passed regulations reducing and limiting the fortification of foods with cholecalciferol, cases ceased to be reported. Similar situations have been found in other countries.

Secondly, it is possible to provide each infant or child with a daily supplement of the vitamin. A dose of 5 ml of standard cod-liver oil, which can also be provided in concentrated form in a capsule, meets the recommended intake of 10 µg. This supplementary intake is a sure and safe way of preventing rickets, but it requires the daily collaboration of the mother. Experience has shown that it is difficult to persuade more than a minority of mothers to give such supplements regularly to their children. In areas where cases of rickets do occur it is very important to educate mothers in the use of the supplement.

After the age of seven, a daily intake of 2.5 µg is recommended, but with reservations. Even if one lives in a country where margarine and butter are not enriched with cholecalciferol, or if one is allergic to eggs and dislikes fatty fish, he can safely go without cod-liver oil by spending half an hour each day walking in the open air during daylight.

Softening of the bones due to a lack of calcium, or *osteomalacia*, is the adult form of rickets. It was formerly seen in women who had repeated pregnancies and lived on very poor diets in large cities where juvenile rickets was rampant. Although this form is now rare, osteomalacia does occur in elderly people, but it is less common than *osteoporosis*, from which it must be distinguished. It is important to ensure that old people who are housebound by infirmities get the recommended amount of cholecalciferol either in their diet or as a vitamin supplement.

International units

Before the chemical nature of vitamin D_3 was known, its vitamin activity was expressed in international units (i.u.). One international unit of vitamin D is equivalent to 0.025 µg of vitamin D_3, or cholecalciferol.

Ascorbic acid (vitamin C)

HISTORY OF SCURVY

Scurvy, the disease arising from the lack of vitamin C, provides an excellent example of how political and economic events may determine the appearance of a nutritional disease. Scurvy was not clearly recognized by physicians in ancient and mediaeval times. Its history begins in 1453, with the sacking of Constantinople by the Turks. As a result, the Venetians lost naval control of the eastern Mediterranean and the overland route between Asia and Europe was blocked. Peppers and other Eastern spices were valuable articles of commerce, for without them the mediaeval European diets were dull and unattractive, especially in the long winter months, when fresh foods were not easily available. This loss stimulated the Portuguese to find a new trade route, and in 1497 Vasco da Gama reached the Malabar coast of southern India after sailing around the Cape of Good Hope. On this long sea voyage he lost 100 men out of his crew of 160 from scurvy. Thereafter, for three hundred years, scurvy was a major factor in determining the success or failure of all sea ventures, whether for purposes of war, trade, or exploration. The discovery that the disease could be prevented by the juice of citrus fruits, especially limes, enabled Captain James Cook, in 1772-75, to make the first journey around the world in which the crew did not develop scurvy and also permitted him to discover Australia. The lime juice stocked on their ships led to the English sailors being known as " limeys " in New York. It also almost doubled the strength of the British navy, because the ships were able to stay at sea for longer than two months without the crews becoming disabled by scurvy.

DESCRIPTION OF SCURVY

The patient with scurvy can usually be recognized easily. The gums are swollen, particularly between the teeth, and bleed easily. Indeed, bleeding occurs readily in all parts of the body, and numerous small haemorrhages may be seen under the skin; large bruises may follow apparently trivial injuries. The big joints, such as the knee or the hip, may appear swollen owing to bleeding into the joint cavity. Sudden death from severe internal haemorrhage and heart failure is always a danger.

Bleeding occurs because of a lack of ascorbic acid, which is necessary to maintain the proteins in the body fluids that bind the cells together. For this purpose collagen is an essential protein, and the formation of new collagen is defective in scurvy. The cells lining the capillaries and small blood vessels become loosened from each other, thus allowing red blood cells to escape from the circulation into the tissue spaces. Defective collagen formation also causes a failure of wounds to heal — a well-known symptom of scurvy.

The body has some capacity for storing the vitamin, mainly in the liver. If the dietary supply of the vitamin is cut off suddenly, this store can meet the needs for a short time, usually for about two months, but if the previous diet has been rich in the vitamin, for as long as six months.

DIETARY SOURCES OF ASCORBIC ACID

The distribution of the vitamin in foods is uneven. Fruits, especially citrus fruits, are rich sources; green vegetables are a useful source, but they contain highly variable amounts, much of which may be lost in preparation and cooking. Root vegetables, such as potatoes, are not a rich source, but since large quantities may be eaten, they can meet requirements. The ascorbic acid content of potatoes goes down in storage and is almost completely destroyed by excessive cooking. Animal products — meat, fish, eggs, and milk — contain only a little. Milk contains sufficient vitamin C for the young infant, but it is easily destroyed by heating. Infantile scurvy was a very important disease at the end of the nineteenth century, when the practice of feeding infants on artificial preparations of cow's milk first became common.

CAUSES AND PREVENTION OF SCURVY TODAY

Scurvy is not an important disease in any part of the world, but doctors everywhere may see occasional cases — usually infants, old people, alcoholics, or dietary cranks. The fact that the medical profession everywhere is still familiar with the disease means that measures to prevent its occurrence continue to be necessary and should not be relaxed. Such measures are in part educational and in part agricultural.

With the decline in breast-feeding associated with urbanization in almost every city of the world, there is an increasing use of artificial milk products, often as the sole source of food for infants from soon after birth. Under these circumstances an increase in cases of infantile scurvy can be expected. Such cases can be prevented by making fruit juice or other supplements of the vitamin readily available.

At the other end of life, declining appetite, immobility and the consequent difficulty in shopping, and poverty each tend to reduce intakes of ascorbic acid. Ensuring old people diets that contain adequate vitamins is now a major responsibility, borne partly by sons and daughters, by religious and other charities, and by local or central government agencies. There is also a widespread need for education in what constitutes a good diet for old people.

In every country, on a national level, agriculture should be planned or directed so that the human food supply provides sufficient vitamin C. In those parts of the world where the rainfall is sufficient and reliable and there is ample sunshine, this should not be difficult. Of course, a very different problem exists in cold countries of the extreme northern and southern hemispheres, as well as in desert or semidesert areas of the tropics and subtropics, because in such areas the diet is likely to provide only a bare margin of safety.

Ascorbic acid is now so cheap and readily available from the chemical industry that it provides the best method of preventing scurvy in an emergency. An ample supply of ascorbic acid should be included in any plans for disaster relief or prevention, as in a military situation, after a flood or earthquake, among political refugees, or on explorations and other expeditions to remote places.

THE RECOMMENDED INTAKE OF ASCORBIC ACID

The recommended intake of 30 mg of ascorbic acid per day can be provided by half an orange or 50 ml of citrus fruit juice; by a good-sized tomato (30 g) or a small helping (50 g) of good-quality leafy vegetables; or by a large helping (120 g) of potatoes, provided that they have not been stored for many months and that the ascorbic acid has not been destroyed by excessive cooking. There are, however, many people who eat smaller amounts of these foods and yet do not suffer from scurvy — who, in fact, appear to be in excellent health. On the contrary, many people take far more than the recommended intake, especially in the U.S.A., where drinking large amounts of fruit juice is a common habit.

The recommended intake is indeed a compromise, albeit a safe and sensible one that makes for good diets. There is adequate evidence from experiments with volunteers, from experimental diets lacking in the vitamin, and from field studies that a daily intake of 10 mg not only provides protection against scurvy, but is indeed sufficient to cure the disease. There have been many claims that higher levels of intake improve health, increase resistance of the body to infections, and enable more rapid recovery from wounds, injuries, and operations, but none of these claims rest on a solid foundation of scientific observation.

The recommended intake, which is at least three times the minimal requirement, provides a large margin of safety — which is important since fruits and vegetables vary so much in ascorbic acid content and losses in cooking and preparation may be considerable. Furthermore, despite the fact that although diets almost totally lacking in fruits and vegetables are consumed by a few people from choice and by many people in all countries because of poverty, a good traditional diet in any country contains a sufficient amount of these foods to provide 30 mg of ascorbic acid per day.

American nutritionists have long made recommendations for very high intakes of ascorbic acid; these have now been reduced, but they still remain substantially above the FAO/WHO recommendation. For other countries the FAO/WHO recommendation, translated into terms of fruits and vegetables, provides a sound basis for national agricultural planning and horticulture on a large scale. Moreover, there must be few villages in the world where the people could not grow more fruits and vegetables if they had the knowledge, especially in view of the many advances in the art and science of gardening; more important, perhaps, is the lack of secure markets for their surplus products. In the growing industrial cities, where fruits and vegetables are often expensive, people find other superficially more attractive but less nutritious foods on which to spend the limited family food budget. The value of fruits and vegetables in the diet is an important topic for teachers of nutrition, home economics, health education, and agriculture.

Thiamine (vitamin B₁)

BERIBERI AND THIAMINE DEFICIENCY

Beriberi, an ancient disease among rice-eating peoples in the East, arises from the consumption of diets containing a high proportion of polished white rice. It exists in three forms. Dry beriberi is a chronic wasting disease, in which neuritis leads to paralysis of the limbs. Wet beriberi is a more acute form of the disease, which causes the whole body to swell from an accumulation of excess water (oedema) and produces disturbances in the circulatory system which may lead to sudden death from heart failure. In a population afflicted by cases of wet and dry beriberi a large number of people are found to be suffering from loss of appetite, malaise, and general weakness, especially in the legs. Such a condition, which greatly reduces work capacity, may persist for months or even years with little variation in the symptoms until suddenly either the dry or wet form of the disease develops. Infantile beriberi is common between the second and fifth months of life in children who are being suckled by mothers subsisting on beriberi-producing diets. Usually an acute disorder, it commonly causes sudden death.

A patient with wet beriberi who is lying in bed breathless, waterlogged, and apparently dying may recover in one or two hours after being given an injection of thiamine — perhaps the most dramatic cure in medicine. Similar dramatic recoveries also occur when an infant with beriberi is given the vitamin; however, the paralysis associated with dry beriberi does not respond to such treatment, although a little improvement may slowly follow after general dietary and other therapy.

Although beriberi was known to the ancient physicians, it did not become an important disease until the introduction of steel rice mills. Then, for fifty years, approximately from 1870 to 1920, it was a dominant disease in the East, affecting in particular the labour forces on plantations and engineering construction works, the police, the prison population, and frequently patients in hospital. India was the only rice-eating country in which beriberi was limited, because in most parts of India it was, and remains, the custom to parboil the paddy in the husk before milling. Parboiling greatly reduces the losses of thiamine and other vitamins which occur in milling.

In the last fifty years beriberi has steadily declined; today it is almost unknown in Tokyo, Hong Kong, Manila, Saigon, Bangkok, Singapore, Djakarta, Kuala Lumpur, and Rangoon — all cities where it was widespread at the beginning of the century. Why beriberi has disappeared from these cities is not immediately obvious. There have been no major changes either in milling practices or in the diets of the people. It is possible, even probable, that the rice is now not quite so finely polished as it formerly was. Also, there has been some general all-round improvement in diets, including greater consumption of pulses and other foods containing thiamine. More important, perhaps, knowledge of the cause of beriberi and of how to prevent it is widespread. Preparations of synthetic thiamine are easily available in towns and cities throughout the East. Although the inhabitants of these cities, as well as of the country areas surrounding them, are clearly getting sufficient thiamine to prevent beriberi, the margin of safety must be small. The situation demands continuing watchful eyes.

Outbreaks of beriberi have occurred among Europeans subsisting on diets based on refined wheat flour — for example, among the British troops besieged by the Turks in Kut-el-Amara in 1916 and among the fishermen of Newfoundland and Labrador in the 1920s. Beriberi is, however, a rare disease in Europe and North America, as well as in Africa and Latin America. In all countries there are individuals in whose diets a large proportion of the energy is provided either by sugar or by alcohol. In many of these diets the supply of thiamine can be only marginally adequate. Indeed, the condition of alcoholic neuritis is clinically indistinguishable from dry beriberi, and both probably arise from the same cause.

DISTRIBUTION OF THIAMINE IN FOODS

All animal and plant tissues depend on thiamine, as it is an essential component of the cell mechanism for the utilization of carbohydrate. Therefore, all natural foods contain thiamine, even if only in small amounts. Plant seeds, however, contain a store that meets the needs of the growing plant embryo; hence, whole cereal grains and pulses are good sources. Yeast is the only very rich natural source. Foods lacking in thiamine are all man-made — refined rice and cereal flours, from which almost all the natural store of the vitamin has been removed by the millers, refined sugar, separated animal and vegetable oils and fats, and alcoholic beverages. None of the thiamine in the yeasts used for fermentation is present in the beers, wines, and spirits that enter normal commerce, although home-brewed beers and country wines may contain significant amounts. Indeed, there are communities in Africa and Latin America which derive the major part of their thiamine from native beers.

The supply of thiamine thus depends on a balance between the intake of natural and processed foods. In rice diets this balance is traditionally and effectively maintained by pulses; thus 25 g of pulse contains sufficient thiamine for utilization of the carbohydrate present in 100 g of rice.

In some countries where the staple food is bread made from highly milled wheat, it is required by law that the flour be enriched with added thiamine. It is also possible to enrich rice grains with thiamine, but the process is technically not so simple as for wheat flour.

THIAMINE REQUIREMENTS

As was indicated above, thiamine is essential for the utilization of carbohydrate in the body. As the carbohydrate is utilized, so is the thiamine. Thiamine requirements are thus closely related to carbohydrate intake. In rice diets, which are usually associated with beriberi, 75 percent or even more of the energy is provided by carbohydrate. If, however, the thiamine content of a diet is related to the total energy content of the diet, rather than only to the energy derived from carbohydrate, the error involved is not large. It has long been customary to express thiamine needs in terms of milligrams per 1 000 kilocalories, as this approach gives practical results. Field studies have shown that all diets associated with beriberi contain less than 0.30 mg/1 000 kcal, and most of them less than 0.25 mg/1 000 kcal. Most persons whose diet provides more than 0.33 mg/1 000 kcal excrete the excess in the urine. The body possesses little ability to store thiamine, and even a person who has previously enjoyed a good diet is liable to develop beriberi in a few weeks if given a beriberi-producing diet. The recommended intake of 0.40 mg/1 000 kcal includes a safety margin designed to cover individual variations. This figure has been used for calculating the recommended thiamine intakes for the various age groups as given in Table 1.

The thiamine requirements of a country are met by any one of the following conditions:

(a) if the staple cereal is not overmilled;

(b) if the staple cereal is fortified with thiamine;

(c) if adequate amounts of alternative foods rich in thiamine (e.g., pulses) are available.

These are matters which must be the concern of central government agencies.

The thiamine requirements of an individual are satisfied if his diet does not contain disproportionate amounts of the following:

(a) refined, unfortified cereal;

(b) refined sugar;

(c) alcohol.

Since these are usually matters of personal choice, nutrition education is important.

Niacin

PELLAGRA AND NIACIN

The discovery of the role of niacin as a vitamin of the B group is closely linked with the story of pellagra. This disease provides another example of how social and economic factors affect the health of man. Pellagra was unknown to physicians of the ancient world and of the Middle Ages. It was first described by the physician G. Casal in Spain in 1730, soon after the introduction of maize into Europe, and was given its name (*pelle*, skin, *agra*, sour) in 1771 by F. Frapolli, an Italian physician. The typical features of the disease, then as now, are increasing weakness and a characteristic skin rash, found only on those surfaces of the body exposed to the sun. It is often marked by severe diarrhoea and mental deterioration. Generations of medical students have remembered pellagra as the disease of the three Ds: dermatitis, diarrhoea, and dementia. In most cases the disease is mild and chronic, the dermatitis recurring each year with the spring sunlight. Patients debilitated and weakened by the diarrhoea often die from infections, and many become inmates of mental asylums.

The disease spread with the cultivation of maize. In the nineteenth century it was common in almost all the European and African countries bordering on the Mediterranean Sea, and it later spread to other African countries. Pellagra had long been present in both North and South America, but it reached epidemic proportions in the South of the U.S.A. after the Civil War, which left in its wake social disruption and poverty, as a result of which many Negro and poor white families had little to eat but maize. The outbreaks were so widespread and severe that most physicians considered the cause to be an infectious agent. It was not until the U.S. Federal Government sent a New York doctor, J. Goldberger, to study the disease that its true nature was determined. He was able to show that the incidence of the disease was closely related to the quality of the diet and that certain foods (e.g., yeast, milk, and meat) were pellagra-preventive and could also be used to treat the disease. Pellagra remained a common major disease in the American South until 1942, when the U.S.A. entered World War II. The consequent full employment greatly reduced poverty, and better wages made the people less dependent on maize. Pellagra disappeared suddenly and has not returned.

Pellagra has declined in all parts of the world. Although isolated cases are often reported from many areas, Africa is probably the only continent in which the disease remains an important public health problem. This is certainly true of South Africa, as many physicians there are well aware. Pellagra still occurs in Egypt as well, although much less frequently than before.

The relation of niacin to pellagra was established when it was isolated from liver extracts and shown to have dramatic curative effects on human cases of pellagra. Both niacinamide (nicotinamide) and niacin (nicotinic acid) function as a vitamin, while nicotine, although chemically related to these substances, does not.

DISTRIBUTION OF NIACIN IN FOODS

Niacin is widely distributed in plant and animal foods, but in most of these it is present in only small amounts. Meats, especially liver, are rich sources, as are whole cereals and pulses. Milling may remove most of the niacin from a cereal, however, in the same way that it removes the thiamine. The discovery of niacin's dramatic effects on pellagra did not explain all the dietary aspects of the disease. In the first place, maize diets consumed by groups in which pellagra was prevalent were shown to provide as much niacin or even more than many poor rice diets which were not associated with pellagra. Secondly, although well known as a preventive and cure for pellagra, milk was found to be a poor source of niacin.

Explanation of the first difficulty appeared with the discovery that in many cereals, and especially in maize, the vitamin is present in a bound form known as niacytin. Since niacytin cannot be broken down by the digestive juices, the niacin in it never becomes available to the tissues of the body. Niacin can, however, be liberated from niacytin when digested with alkalis. This probably explains why Mexicans who eat tortillas are relatively free of pellagra. In making tortillas the maize flour is treated with limewater before cooking; thus the niacin is released from the niacytin and made fully available to the body tissues.

Explanation of the second difficulty followed the discovery that niacin can be manufactured in the body from tryptophan, an essential amino acid. The process is not very effective, however, as the body has many other uses for tryptophan. In fact, about 60 mg of tryptophan is required to produce 1 mg of niacin. Milk is a very rich source of tryptophan and therefore has pellagra-preventive properties, although it contains little niacin. In discussion of niacin requirements it is usual to express the niacin content of foods in terms of niacin equivalents. By definition a niacin equivalent is equal to 1 mg of niacin or 60 mg of tryptophan. Milk has a high value in niacin equivalents.

NIACIN REQUIREMENTS

Niacinamide (nicotinamide) has an essential role in the oxidative mechanisms by which the chemical energy present in the molecules of carbohydrate, fat, and protein is liberated and made available to the cells of the body for work or as heat. It is reasonable to relate requirement to energy intake, which, as in the case of thiamine, is expressed in milligrams per 1 000 kcal. The recommended requirement is based largely on studies of human volunteers on diets low in niacin equivalents. It was found that when the diet was improved so as to contain 5.5 niacin equivalents per 1 000 kcal, the subjects excreted large amounts of a derivative of niacinamide (nicotinamide) in their urine. This dietary intake was seen to meet the requirements of these volunteers, and a safety margin for individual variation was added, to arrive at the recommended daily intake of 6.6 niacin equivalents per 1 000 kcal. This figure was used in calculating the recommended niacin intakes for the various age groups given in Table 1.

To raise the niacin content of the diet of a community, it is possible to fortify the staple cereal with the vitamin. Some countries fortify refined cereals, which in themselves are low in niacin and, perhaps, also in tryptophan. However, considering the niacin equivalent per 1 000 kcal in most mixed diets, it appears that the need for such action is not common.

Wide experience in maize-eating countries shows that the presence or absence of pellagra is closely related to the economic state of the community. If this improves, more meat and milk are consumed, the niacin intake increases, and pellagra disappears. Providing sufficient employment and a good market for agricultural and other products appears to be the most effective means of ensuring that the recommended intake is met.

Riboflavine

The extract first called vitamin B_2 was known to contain a mixture of growth-promoting factors, one of which was isolated and shown to be a yellow pigment which was named riboflavine. Riboflavine is still sometimes referred to as vitamin B_2, but this is not strictly correct. Riboflavine, like niacinamide (nicotinamide), has an essential role in the oxidative mechanisms in the cells of all body tissues.

DISTRIBUTION OF RIBOFLAVINE IN FOODS

Riboflavine is so widely distributed that it is found in most foods. As has already been indicated, yeast is a rich source. Meat, eggs, and fish are good sources. Milk contains useful amounts, but these depend, as in the case of retinol, on the diet of the animal producing the milk. Green leafy vegetables vary greatly, but some are rich in riboflavine, as are most pulses. Whole-cereal grains contain useful amounts, but these are removed in milling, which means that highly milled cereals contain very little. It is, however, the only vitamin present in significant amounts in beer. Indeed, beer drinkers may be interested to know that one litre daily almost meets the recommended intake.

RIBOFLAVINE DEFICIENCY

Soon after 1935, when riboflavine became available for therapeutic trials, it was found that small doses rapidly cured certain conditions common in malnourished people — for example, sores at the angles of the mouth (angular stomatitis); sore, swollen, and chapped lips (cheilosis); swollen, fissured, and painful tongues (glossitis); and redness and congestion at the edges of the cornea of the eye. All of these conditions are common, especially in children in tropical areas where the dietary supply of meat, milk, fruits, and vegetables is poor. The same conditions are sometimes seen in persons of all ages, but particularly in elderly people, in the U.K. and many other well-fed countries. There, these conditions seldom respond to treatment with riboflavine or other vitamins, and it is generally recognized that they can arise from causes unrelated to the diet. Riboflavine deficiency should be diagnosed only when one or another of these conditions is shown to respond to treatment with the vitamin.

Unlike all the other vitamins discussed in this handbook, riboflavine deficiency is not the cause of any severe or major disease of man. Nevertheless, diets which lead to beriberi, pellagra, scurvy, keratomalacia, or nutritional megaloblastic anaemia are likely to be poor in riboflavine. Riboflavine deficiency probably often contributes to disorders and disabilities from which patients with these diseases suffer.

RECOMMENDED INTAKES OF RIBOFLAVINE

As for thiamine and niacin, the recommended intakes are usually related to the dietary energy intake. Clinical evidence of deficiency in subjects on experimental diets has not been found when the diet has provided more than 0.25 mg/1 000 kcal, but significant amounts of riboflavine do not appear in the urine until intakes of 0.50 mg/ 1 000 kcal are reached. Dietary studies indicate that signs of riboflavine deficiency are likely to arise when the individual daily intake falls to 0.50 mg. On the basis of these considerations a riboflavine intake of 0.60 mg/1 000 kcal is recommended. This provides a reasonable margin for individual variability.

In places where the diet is likely to be deficient in riboflavine, the presence or absence of clinical evidence of the deficiency often depends on seasonal variations in the quality of the diet. Often an apparently small increase in the intake of one or two foods is followed by a rapid disappearance of the clinical signs. To ensure satisfactory intakes of riboflavine, it is best to try to improve the all-round quality of the diet, rather than to concentrate on any one source.

Cereals can be fortified with riboflavine, but this inevitably makes them (especially rice) yellow and therefore unacceptable. Medicinal preparations of riboflavine are readily available and can be used to supplement the diets of pregnant women or in other cases where it may be thought necessary.

Folates

In 1931, while working in a maternity hospital in Bombay, Dr. Lucy Wills found that many of the mothers were suffering from a severe type of anaemia. This, like Addisonian anaemia, was megaloblastic, but the patients improved when given extracts of yeast, whereas they did not respond to the partially purified liver extracts then used to treat Addisonian anaemia (see the discussion of pernicious anaemia under cyanocobalamin).

Subsequent work showed that the factor in yeast which was effective in curing Dr. Wills's patients was a vitamin or, rather, a group of chemically related vitamins known as folates. Most foods contain some folates, but only leafy vegetables and a few flesh foods are rich sources. The term folate comes from the Latin word *folium*, meaning leaf. For many years folic acid has been established as a reliable remedy for a form of megaloblastic anaemia that is common in India and in other tropical countries and occurs occasionally throughout the world.

There is still real difficulty, however, in assessing the folate content of foods and in making recommendations for dietary intake. First of all, the methods used for determining the folate content of foods do not all give consistent results; secondly, there is still some uncertainty regarding the extent to which the different forms of folate can be absorbed from the intestine and made available. Most people in the U.K. and the U.S.A., where dietary deficiency is uncommon, eat diets providing 100-200 μg of free folate per day; but in many countries diets providing only 50 μg are common. The recommended daily intake has been set at 200 μg for adults, which appears a safe and sensible recommendation, although future work may prove the target to have been set too high. To reach it, the consumption of green vegetables and meat in many countries would have to increase greatly.

Dr. Wills's original patients with megaloblastic anaemia were almost all pregnant women. There is no doubt that in some way, as yet unknown, pregnancy greatly increases the requirements of folate — at least in some women. Although megaloblastic anaemia during pregnancy which responds to folate is not common in prosperous countries, it does continue to occur. Furthermore, the anaemia may be severe and in some cases fatal in the absence of treatment with the vitamin. Therefore, the recommended intake for pregnant women is doubled to 400 μg per day. Folate can be readily provided in medicinal form. Tablets containing 100 μg of folic acid, together with iron, are available, and many obstetricians and nutritionists recommend that such tablets should be taken three times a day by all women during the last three months of pregnancy.

Folate deficiency, like vitamin B_{12} deficiency, may accompany disease of the alimentary tract and lead to megaloblastic anaemia. Since human milk and other milks are not rich in folate, the newborn infant is probably partly dependent on a store in the liver laid down from supplies provided by the mother before birth. If birth is premature, this store may be small and folate may be required to correct anaemia.

Cyanocobalamin (vitamin B_{12})

In 1849 Thomas Addison, a physician working at Guy's Hospital in London, described a form of anaemia, occurring mostly in middle-aged and elderly patients, which progressed slowly and ended with the death of the patient in two to five years. So inevitable was its course that the disease was known as pernicious anaemia. There was no hope for victims of this disease until 1926, when G.R. Minot at the Harvard Medical School showed that it could be cured by eating large amounts of liver. W.B. Castle, a colleague of Minot and his successor in the chair of medicine at Harvard, found that this form of anaemia was due to the lack of a substance present in liver and meat.

It was ascertained, however, that pernicious anaemia stemmed not from a dietary deficiency, but from a failure of the stomach to secrete an " intrinsic factor " essential for the absorption of the dietary " extrinsic factor " from the small intestine. Subsequently this latter factor was isolated from liver and shown to be a substance containing cobalt, which is now called cyanocobalamin or vitamin B_{12}. Some patients with pernicious anaemia have been kept in good health by treatment with injections of as little as one millionth of a gram (1 μg) daily. Although the nature of the "intrinsic factors" secreted by the stomach remains for the most part a mystery, victims of pernicious anaemia stay in good health with their blood remaining normal provided they receive an injection of the vitamin every two or three weeks. Hence, the old name of the disease is now inapt, and it is better to refer to it as Addisonian anaemia. This is one of the great success stories of modern medicine. However, as has already been stated, whereas Addisonian anaemia does not normally arise from a dietary lack, only recently it has been shown that a dietary deficiency of cyanocobalamin, or vitamin B_{12}, may be a contributory cause of anaemia.

CHANGES IN THE BLOOD CAUSED BY CYANOCOBALAMIN DEFICIENCY

The red cells in Addisonian anaemia are characteristically larger than normal and irregular in size and shape. Normal red blood cells develop in the bone marrow from large primitive cells which contain a nucleus but lack the pigment haemoglobin. Microscopic examination of the bone marrow of patients with Addisonian anaemia shows that the disease arises from a failure of these primitive cells to develop and mature into normal red cells. This type of anaemia is said to be megaloblastic.

DIETARY SOURCES AND RECOMMENDED INTAKE OF CYANOCOBALAMIN

Plants cannot manufacture this vitamin and do not utilize it. It is present, however, in many moulds and can, in fact, be prepared easily and cheaply as a by-product of the process for making the antibiotic streptomycin. Very small amounts are present in all animal tissues, so all foods of animal origin contain at least traces. The only rich source is liver, the organ in which a store of the vitamin is maintained. This store depletes slowly and in man is sufficient to last for twelve months or longer. Indeed, the presence of a store of the vitamin accounts for the slow and insidious course of Addisonian anaemia.

In the U.S.A. an analysis of diets classified as high cost, low cost, and poor showed that these supplied 31, 16, and 2.7 μg of vitamin B_{12} daily, whereas patients with Addisonian anaemia can be kept in good health on 1 µg per day. Experiments on patients and healthy subjects indicate that daily losses of the vitamin range from 0.25 µg to nearly 1 µg. From this evidence a recommended intake of 2 µg per day has been prescribed for the normal adult.

Dietary deficiency of cyanocobalamin

The dietary intake falls below the recommended amount in many people living on poor diets which are for practical purposes vegetarian. Vegetarianism is, of course, common amongst Hindus in India and elsewhere, but most of them drink milk and some eat eggs and fish. Yet, for large numbers of Hindus the intake of animal foods and therefore of vitamin B_{12} no doubt falls short of the recommended amount. Some degree of megaloblastic anaemia is widespread in India, and severe megaloblastic anaemia is much more frequent there than in Europe, although folate deficiency rather than cyanocobalamin deficiency is perhaps the most important cause. Very low individual intakes of the vitamin have also been recorded in surveys carried out in Peru and North Africa.

The story of vitamin B_{12} is not yet complete, but the facts already known lend support to all programmes designed to improve animal husbandry and to increase the supply and consumption of animal protein. Vitamin B_{12} deficiency is a not uncommon consequence of many diseases and surgical operations on the stomach and small intestine. These are matters of importance to the medical profession, but need not concern us here.

5. CALCIUM

The skeleton of an adult man contains about 1.2 kg of calcium, which in the form of calcium phosphate constitutes most of the hard structure of bone. This is laid down on a bed, or matrix, of protein, of which the human skeleton contains about 2 kg. By the age of 20 the bones have ceased to grow in length, but they probably thicken and become more dense up to the age of 25; thereafter they slowly waste and become thinner. With advancing age the bones become fragile and may break more easily. If this process is accelerated, it gives rise to the disease known as osteoporosis, common in old people in all countries, which may cause great pain and eventual disability.

CALCIUM IN FOODS

As calcium is present in the tissues of plants and animals, all natural human foods contain small amounts of the element, while processed foods, such as refined sugar and extracted oils and fats, contain none. Milk and milk products and fish consumed whole are very rich in calcium. Ragi (*Eleucine coracana*), a millet, contains 300-400 mg of calcium per 100 g.

GROWTH AND MAINTENANCE OF BONE

In general, the size of adults is related to the amount of milk they drank as children; in countries where there is little milk the people are usually small. It therefore seemed sensible to attribute failure to grow and the corresponding small skeleton to a lack of dietary calcium; however, much recent work has shown this to be wrong. Samples of bones taken from persons whose previous diet has been either rich or poor in calcium have been shown to have the same chemical composition and to contain similar amounts of the mineral. The bones of people whose diet is low in calcium appear to be of normal density when examined by X ray and do not fracture more easily than normal. Milk promotes the growth of the skeleton by providing protein for the formation of the matrix on which the minerals are deposited. If the diet is defective, this matrix is formed slowly, growth is delayed, and the adult bones tend to be small. Nevertheless, all human diets appear to provide enough calcium to complete the mineralization of such matrix as is formed, and such small bones are therefore of good quality.

The factors that determine the speed at which the bones waste, or atrophy, after the age of 25 are imperfectly understood. The process may be accelerated by insufficient physical activity and by disturbances in the balance of the endocrine glands, but there is no convincing evidence that the level of dietary calcium modifies the process. Orthodox medical opinion holds that both the growth and atrophy of bone proceed at rates which are independent of the calcium in the diet.

If it takes 25 years to form a mature skeleton containing 1.2 kg of calcium, then, on the average, some 130 mg of calcium must have been retained daily during this period. In addition, bone, once formed, is not permanent, but is slowly renewed; in an adult this probably involves the turnover of some 700 mg of calcium daily. Much of this calcium can be utilized again for bone formation, but some is lost in the urine. The output of calcium in the urine varies widely in individuals, ranging from 50 to 300 mg per day, but the amount excreted is little affected by the level of intake. At all ages enough calcium must be absorbed in the small intestine to make good this normal loss, and in childhood and youth additional amounts are needed to provide for growth.

CALCIUM ABSORPTION

Normally, intestinal absorption of calcium is precisely regulated to meet these needs. The control mechanism is not properly understood, but it is surely dependent on vitamin D. If the supply of this vitamin is inadequate, calcium absorption is impaired and the reserve of calcium in the bones is drawn upon. As a result the bones become soft and the condition of osteomalacia arises. Osteomalacia may also follow upon chronic disease of the small intestine.

Calcium can only be absorbed from the intestine when it is in solution. For example, insoluble calcium salts readily form in the intestine with phytic acid, oxalic acid, and fatty acids. Of these, phytic acid, present in cereals, is the most important. If persons living on diets containing ample milk and rich in calcium are transferred suddenly to a low calcium diet containing a high proportion of cereals, they are unable to absorb the calcium, most of which is lost in the faeces as calcium phytate. Such persons go into a negative calcium balance. It was this observation that was responsible in part for former recommendations of high calcium intakes. Further experiments have shown, however, that a subject who is kept on a low calcium, high cereal diet adapts after a short period, usually a few weeks, and is able to digest the calcium phytate and to absorb and utilize the calcium. He then returns to a state of equilibrium on the low calcium intake.

CALCIUM REQUIREMENTS

The FAO/WHO Expert Group on Calcium Requirements met in 1961. At that time many authorities recommended high intakes of calcium for the reasons indicated above. Furthermore, dietary calcium deficiency was held to be widespread in the world, and a policy for extensive fortification of cereals and other foods with calcium had been advocated. On the evidence then available it took courage to state that high intakes of calcium were unnecessary and that requirements could be met with less than half the customary intakes in most European countries and in North America. Since the publication of the report, much new evidence has supported the position taken by the Expert Group, which expressed its recommended intakes as ranges — for example, 400-500 mg daily for adults. Recent work has justified the use of the low figures in the ranges for assessing the adequacy of diets, and these are given in Table 1.

PREGNANCY AND LACTATION

The growth of a full-term foetus requires about 30 g of calcium, most of which must be made available in the last trimester of pregnancy. A nursing mother may release as much as 300 mg of calcium daily in her milk. The recommended intake of 1 000-1 200 mg per day during the last trimester of pregnancy and lactation is ample to meet these needs. In fact, in countries throughout the world many women with only a small supply of milk in their diet have gone through several successful pregnancies and lactations on much lower calcium intakes. Nevertheless, the high recommended intakes are compatible with the best system of diet that can be given to mothers, although, unfortunately, such advice is not always practical.

CALCIUM EXCESS

Normally, the small intestine acts as an effective control and prevents an excess of calcium from being absorbed. However, a breakdown of this control raises the level of calcium in the blood and leads to pathological calcification of the kidneys and other internal organs. This may occur in infants who have usually been fed on artificial foods fortified with excessive amounts of vitamin D and calcium.

Everywhere in the world, urinary stones occur occasionally in otherwise healthy persons. Such individuals usually have a high output of urinary calcium, to which in some cases high dietary calcium may contribute. In several areas of the world, urinary stones are notably common, though the dietary intake of calcium in these areas is usually low; despite much research the reason for this remains a mystery.

6. IRON

The body of an adult human contains 3 to 4 g of iron, of which more than two thirds is present in haemoglobin, the pigment of the red blood cells. The rest of the iron in the body is present as a reserve store in the liver and, to a lesser extent, in the kidney, spleen, and other organs. Despite the very small amounts in the body, iron is one of the most important elements in nutrition and of fundamental importance to life. Iron is a component of haemoglobin, myoglobin, the cytochromes, catalase, peroxidase, and certain other enzyme systems. As a part of these haeme complexes and metallo enzymes, it serves important functions in oxygen transport and cellular respiration.

The red blood cells and the pigment within are broken down and replaced every 120 days, but the liberated iron is not excreted, as most of it is utilized to form new haemoglobin. The total daily iron loss of an adult man weighing 65 kg is about 0.9 mg.

ABSORPTION OF IRON FROM FOOD

Absorption of iron can take place from the stomach and throughout the whole of the small intestine; however, the greatest absorption occurs in the upper part of the small intestine. Only 10 percent of the iron present in cereals, vegetables, and pulses, excluding soybeans, is absorbed. Absorption of iron from other foods is slightly higher — for instance, 30 percent from meat, 20 percent from soybean, and 15 percent from fish. For estimating the absorption of iron in diets, a weighted upper value of 20 percent has therefore been taken as the percentage of iron absorbed from foods of animal and soybean origin.

Ascorbic acid, sulphydryl groups, and similar reducing substances facilitate the absorption of ingested iron, but the mechanism is not well understood. Iron absorption increases when there is increased haemoglobin synthesis — for example, following haemorrhages or resulting from anaemia and haemopoetic abnormalities. Absorption also increases during growth and pregnancy. Phytic acid and an excess of phosphates may impair iron absorption, because of the formation of insoluble iron salts which pass through the intestinal tract without being absorbed.

EXCRETION OF IRON

Absorbed iron is lost only by exfoliation from the alimentary, urinary, and respiratory tracts and by dermal and hair losses. The bulk of ingested iron is excreted in the faeces. Urinary iron excretion is so small as to be negligible, with mean values of approximately 0.1 mg or less per day. Only in cases of renal diseases, particularly nephrosis, does urinary excretion of iron become appreciable.

Recent studies of the loss of radioisotopic iron by men living in several countries suggest that the combined losses by all routes are of the order of 1 mg per day or less. In women, with smaller body sizes, this probably falls to about 0.8 mg per day, but they have the added burden of iron losses associated with the blood loss of menstruation. In industrialized countries, blood donation represents another major form of iron loss. Pathological bleeding (hookworm infections, bleeding ulcers, etc.) can also be an important source of iron loss.

IRON REQUIREMENTS

Only very small amounts of iron are lost from the body, mostly in the cells, or shed from the skin and the epithelial surfaces lining the alimentary and urinary tracts. This daily iron loss in an adult man weighing 65 kg has been estimated as 0.91 mg. Since the mean absorption of dietary iron is only 10-20 percent, a daily allowance of 6-9 mg will cover the needs of an adult man.

In addition to the physiological losses of iron, women who are menstruating normally lose up to 2 mg per day in the menstrual blood. Hence the iron requirements of an adult woman are much higher than those of an adult man.

In the case of infants the iron requirements should not only compensate for basal iron losses, but also provide for an increase in haemoglobin mass and in the iron content of body tissues associated with growth. A normal full-term infant is born with adequate stores of iron and, if breast-fed, shows little or no increase in body iron before the end of the fourth month. During this time there is, instead, a redistribution of iron between a decreasing haemoglobin mass and an increasing tissue iron mass. During the succeeding eight months the estimated body iron increments are about 0.5 mg per day, while the estimated daily losses are also about 0.5 mg, which means that the total daily requirement of absorbed iron is about 1.0 mg. The body iron content of a one-year-old infant should be 400 mg.

In pregnant women iron is required not only to replace basal physiological losses, but also to allow for expansion of the red cell mass and to provide for the needs of the foetus and placenta. The net cost of pregnancy per se is 565 mg of iron. The iron secreted in breast milk has been estimated to be 0.25 mg per day, and an additional requirement of 1-2 mg of iron daily will meet the demands of lactation. The increased requirements of iron during pregnancy and lactation can easily be offset by the normal additional needs for menstruation. Since there is a cessation of menstruation during pregnancy and early lactation, the allowances for nonpregnant and nonlactating women of childbearing age suffice during pregnancy and lactation. The recommended intakes of iron for different age groups are given in Table 1.

IRON DEFICIENCY

An inadequate dietary intake of iron by growing children, by adolescent girls, or by women, especially during pregnancy and in lactation, will produce nutritional anaemia, characterized by a decrease in the amount of haemoglobin and by small, pale-red blood cells, depleted iron stores, and a plasma iron content of less than 40 mg/100 ml. The number of red blood cells may also be reduced, but not as markedly as the haemoglobin content.

If the pregnant woman has an insufficient intake of iron, the newborn infant, in turn, will have a relatively low store of iron, causing anaemia to develop early in the first year of life. Anaemia during infancy, a frequent phenomenon, is closely related to the body stores of iron at birth. It is especially common in premature infants and twins, because in such circumstances the body reserves of iron cannot be built up to desirable levels.

Many adolescent girls, even today, select a poor diet, to indulge the whims of a freakish appetite or to maintain ill-advised reduction regimens, with resultant anaemia. Thus it is necessary to continually emphasize the fact that during adolescence there is an accelerated demand for iron to satisfy the still-increasing blood volume as well as compensate for losses through menstruation.

Iron-deficiency anaemia is a medical and public health problem of primary importance, causing few deaths but contributing seriously to the weakness, ill health, and substandard performance of millions of people.

INTAKES OF IRON

As iron is widely distributed in all foodstuffs, the diets consumed by a majority of the world's population provide more than adequate amounts of iron. Approximately equal contributions to the daily iron intake are made by meat, poultry, and fish; whole grain or enriched cereals and breads; and green or yellow vegetables. Certain fruits — peaches, apricots, prunes, grapes, and raisins — are excellent sources of available iron if they are eaten fairly often. While fruits and other vegetables, including potatoes, contain lesser concentrations of iron, the daily intake of these food groups may be sufficiently high to account for important additions to iron intake.

Normal mixed human diets of good quality contain approximately 12-15 mg of iron, of which slightly more than 1 mg is absorbed. This amount is adequate for adult males, but it is inadequate for adolescent girls or women on diets of a less than 10 percent calorie content from animal foods; for this reason the iron requirements for the latter have been set by the FAO/WHO Expert Committee at 24 and 28 mg per day, respectively. Obviously it is difficult to design a diet which normally contains this amount of iron, and it is to be expected that under these circumstances a certain proportion of adolescent girls and menstruating women will not be able to meet their requirement without recourse to iron supplementation.

In certain affluent countries, notably in the U.S.A., where populations consume highly refined foods, normal diets have been found to contain 6-7 mg of iron, a level which is not high enough to satisfy the requirements. The iron levels in such diets can be improved by fortification. The availability of iron added to foods is affected by the form of iron added, the nature of the vehicle, and the quality of other dietary constituents. Most of the evidence suggests that ferrous sulphate, now being used in certain fortification programmes, is among the most available forms.

The American Medical Association's Council of Foods and Nutrition has recently reiterated its previous conclusion that it is in the public interest to increase the iron content of enriched wheat flour, bread, buns, and rolls as proposed by the U.S. Food and Drug Administration.

7. IODINE

Iodine is an essential nutrient for man because it is an integral component of the thyroid hormones thyroxine and triiodothyronine, both of which have important metabolic roles. One of the factors affecting the output of thyroid hormones by the thyroid gland is iodine availability. In the absence of sufficient iodine the gland attempts to compensate for the deficiency by increasing its secretory activity, and this causes the gland to enlarge. This condition is known as simple, or endemic, goitre.

Endemic goitre of varying degrees is found among certain population groups whose sources of dietary iodine are limited. Foods grown on iodine-poor soil contain insufficient iodine to meet human needs. Endemic goitre does not occur when the adult iodine intake ranges upwards from 0.075 mg per day. Dietary iodine absorbed from the small intestine follows two main pathways within the body. Approximately 30 percent is removed by the thyroid gland and used for synthesis of thyroid hormones; the remainder is excreted in the urine.

The optimum daily requirement of iodine is 0.14 mg for an adult man and 0.10 mg for an adult woman. Growing children and pregnant or lactating women may need more. The need for iodine increases in pregnancy because the foetus must derive its iodine requirement and reserve from the mother. Maternal iodide is lost during lactation through secretion in the milk, so the minimum iodine requirement increases to almost one and a half times normal.

Among natural foods the best sources of iodine are sea foods and vegetables grown on iodine-rich soils. Dairy products and eggs may be good sources if the producing animals have access to iodine-enriched rations. Most cereal grains, legumes, and roots have a low iodine content. Of the various methods that have been proposed for assuring an adequate iodine intake, especially among populations in iodine-poor regions, the use of iodized salt has thus far proved to be the most successful and therefore the most widely adopted method. Commercial iodized salt contains 0.01 percent potassium iodide or iodate. Assuming that the average adult uses 6-7 g of salt daily, the iodine intake amounts to 0.48 mg, or more than twice the normal requirement, thus providing amply for sufficient reserves.

8. FLUORINE

Fluorine is normally present in the bones and teeth, and a proper intake of this element is essential for maximum resistance to dental caries, or decay. For these reasons fluorine is considered an essential nutrient. The beneficial effect of fluorine in the prevention of dental caries is particularly evident during infancy and early childhood and persists through adult life.

The precise mechanism by which fluorine inhibits the development of dental caries is not known. Incorporated into tooth enamel during the formative period, fluorine apparently reduces the solubility of this enamel in the acids produced by bacteria.

INTAKES OF FLUORIDE

Fluorine is widely but unevenly distributed in nature. It is found in many foods, but sea foods and tea are the most significant dietary sources. An average daily diet provides 0.25 to 0.35 mg of fluorine. In addition, the average adult may ingest 1.0-1.5 mg daily from drinking and cooking water that contains 1 ppm of fluorine. For children 1-12 years old, water may contribute anywhere from 0.4 to 1.1 mg of fluorine per day.

Fluoridation of water supplies

Fluoridation of water supplies in order to bring the concentration of fluoride to 1 ppm has proved to be a safe, economical, and efficient way to reduce tooth decay — a highly important public health measure in areas where natural water supplies do not contain this amount. Extensive medical and public health studies have clearly demonstrated the safety and nutritional advantages that result from fluoridation of water supplies, although the subject is very liable to produce intense outbursts of irrational emotion at the local government level in many developed countries.

FLUORIDE EXCESS

The fluoride content of water increases, sometimes excessively, when it passes through rocks and through soils of certain composition. Use of such water supplies leads to dental fluorosis, characterized by mottling of the enamel of the teeth. This condition is endemic in a number of communities where the natural water supply contains more than 2 ppm of fluoride. The fluoride content of such water can be reduced by ion-exchange treatment.

9. OTHER TRACE ELEMENTS ESSENTIAL FOR HUMAN NUTRITION *

Trace elements — other than iron, iodine, and fluorine — which are reported to have beneficial effects in human subjects are zinc, magnesium, copper, chromium, selenium, cobalt, and molybdenum. Deficiencies of most of these elements have been reported in human diets.

ZINC

The presence of zinc (Zn) in living organisms and its role as an essential nutrient have long been recognized. Since zinc is an integral part of carbonic anhydrase and many other highly purified enzymes, it is thus of importance in protein and carbohydrate metabolism.

Lack of zinc in human diets has been studied in detail in Egypt and Iran. Growth failure and sexual infantilism are reported to result from this deficiency. The major constituent of the diet of individuals in these areas is an unleavened bread prepared from low-extraction wheat flour. The phytate present in the flour limits the availability of zinc in these diets, with the result that the requirements of the element are not satisfied. Zinc-responsive growth failure has also been observed in young children from middle-class homes in the U.S.A. who consume less than an ounce of meat per day.

The zinc requirement for an adult male, derived factorially, is 2.2 mg per day. The amounts of dietary zinc needed to meet requirements vary with the composition of the diet and the availability of the element. If the availability of Zn is 10 percent, the amount of dietary zinc needed daily to meet the requirement would be 22 mg. Growing children and pregnant and lactating women need more.

---

* Discussed by the WHO Expert Committee on Trace Elements in Human Nutrition in 1973 (*Wld Hlth Org. techn. Rep. Ser.*, No. 532, 1973).

Animal foodstuffs are dependable sources of zinc. Beef, pork, and lamb may contain 20-60 µg/g, and milk 3-5 µg/g. Fish and other sea foods contain more than 15 µg/g. Whole cereals are also rich sources of zinc, but appreciable amounts are lost during milling.

MAGNESIUM

The adult human body contains approximately 20-25 g of magnesium (Mg). Despite the relatively large amounts present and demonstrations that magnesium is an essential nutrient for experimental animals, concrete data indicating its role in human nutrition have been presented only recently. Magnesium is known to be required for the activity of a great many enzymes, particularly those concerned with oxidative phosphorylation.

Magnesium deficiency in humans occurs in such conditions as chronic malabsorption syndromes, acute diarrhoea, chronic renal failure, chronic alcoholism, and protein-calorie malnutrition. Symptoms attributed to magnesium deficiency include emotional lability and irritability, tetany, hyperreflexia, and occasionally hyporeflexia.

Adult magnesium requirements have been estimated to lie between 200 and 300 mg per day. An intake of 300 mg daily has been found to maintain a positive balance in women. Estimates of magnesium requirements are based on extremely limited information regarding the absorption, metabolism, and excretion of this nutrient; accordingly, the allowances proposed must be regarded as provisional.

Magnesium is widely distributed in plants. Meat and viscera are rich sources of the element. Milk is a relatively poor source. In a mixed diet containing abundant animal products, magnesium appears to be 30-40 percent available.

COPPER

Copper (Cu) is a component of the enzymes tyrosinase and uricase and is probably associated with other oxidation-reduction enzyme systems. It is believed that copper facilitates the absorption of iron, and it appears to play a role in the synthesis of iron into haemoglobin and cytochrome molecules, but the exact mechanism for this haematopoetic role has not been established.

Copper deficiency has never been reported in adults, although cases of moderate to severe anaemia responsive to copper and iron therapy have been reported in infants. Such subjects manifest pallor, retarded growth, and oedema and suffer from anorexia. Low levels of iron and copper in the serum are other diagnostic features.

A realistic allowance of copper for infants and young children, incorporating a desirable margin of safety, is 80 µg/kg per day. It is probable that 40 µg per kilogram of body weight per day is adequate for older children, and that approximately 30 µg per kilogram daily is sufficient for adults.

Copper is widely distributed in foodstuffs, and a diet of even mediocre quality contains 2-3 mg per day, enough to meet the requirements of man. The richest sources of dietary copper are liver, kidney, shellfish, nuts, raisins, and dried legumes. Milk is a poor source of the element. Homogenized cow's milk contains from 0.015 to 1.18 mg of copper per litre, much less on the average than the 0.6 to 1.05 mg present in a litre of human milk.

CHROMIUM

There is some evidence that chromium (Cr) is an essential nutrient for man. Investigations of the relationship of this element to carbohydrate metabolism are suggestive of its possible role in human nutrition.

Chromium deficiency in man is evidenced by (a) impairment of oral or intravenous glucose tolerance, (b) low tissue concentrations, and (c) a low concentration in the urine.

Absorption of trivalent chromium in man, just as in the rat, may vary from less than 1 percent to 10 or 25 percent. The availability of chromium depends upon its chemical nature in foodstuffs. Dietary intakes varying from 20-50 µg per day are required to compensate for the loss of the element through the urine.

Chromium is present in lower concentrations in vegetable foods than it is in animal foods. Intakes of the element can vary significantly, from 5 to over 100 µg daily. It is present in significant amounts in drinking water.

SELENIUM

Although the need for selenium (Se) seems to be adequately documented for laboratory and farm animals, no corresponding deficiency is known in man. There are, however, reports suggesting that selenium deficiency may be a complicating factor in certain types of protein-calorie malnutrition in children. It has been claimed on the basis of animal experiments that high levels of selenium promote dental caries, and there is some evidence that the same may be true for humans.

Sufficient evidence is not available for the establishment of human requirements.

COBALT

The discovery, in 1948, that vitamin B_{12} (cyanocobalamin) contains 4 percent cobalt (Co) proved this element to be an essential nutrient for man. Cobalt is present in many foods, in cooking utensils, and even in the atmosphere — at least in industrial cities. A deficiency of cobalt in ruminants results in impaired growth, listlessness, progressive emaciation, and varying degrees of anorexia.

Cobalt is readily absorbed in the human intestinal tract, but most of the absorbed material is excreted in the urine; very little of the element is retained. The tained cobalt serves no physiological function since human tissue cannot synthesize vitamin B_{12}. There is no known human requirement for the element, except for that contained in vitamin B_{12}.

The subject of human requirements of vitamin B_{12} was discussed earlier (see page 46).

MOLYBDENUM

Evidence that molybdenum (Mo) is an essential trace element is based on the fact that it is part of the molecular structure of two enzymes, xanthine oxidase and aldehyde oxidase. Diets low in molybdenum adversely affect growth in small animals and depress the activity of xanthine oxidase. There is no evidence, however, to suggest that a low molybdenum intake results in clinical manifestations in man.

Balance studies in human adults have shown that molybdenum equilibrium or a slight positive balance may be maintained if the diet provides 2 μg molybdenum per kilogram of body weight daily. This figure can be tentatively suggested as the requirement for humans.

CONCLUSION

The recommended intakes of nutrients given in Table 1 are based on the findings of contemporary nutritional science. New knowledge may allow some of the recommendations to be fixed more precisely, but it is unlikely that major changes will be necessary. When translated into terms of local foods, the figures can certainly be used as a practical guide for agricultural planning in all countries. It is hoped that the text illustrates their meaning, thus facilitating the task of planning for increased food production, which is so necessary in all countries, especially those in which a large population growth is anticipated.

TABLES

TABLE 1. — RECOMM

Age	Body weight	Energy (1)		Protein (1, 2)	Vitamin A (3, 4)	Vita D (5,
	kilo-grams	kilo-calories	mega-joules	grams	micro-grams	mic gra
Children						
< 1	7.3	820	3.4	14	300	10
1-3	13.4	1 360	5.7	16	250	10
4-6	20.2	1 830	7.6	20	300	10
7-9	28.1	2 190	9.2	25	400	2
Male adolescents						
10-12	36.9	2 600	10.9	30	575	2
13-15	51.3	2 900	12.1	37	725	2
16-19	62.9	3 070	12.8	38	750	2
Female adolescents						
10-12	38.0	2 350	9.8	29	575	2
13-15	49.9	2 490	10.4	31	725	2
16-19	54.4	2 310	9.7	30	750	2
Adult man						
(moderately active) ...	65.0	3 000	12.6	37	750	2
Adult woman						
(moderately active) ...	55.0	2 200	9.2	29	750	2
Pregnancy						
(later half)		+350	+1.5	38	750	10
Lactation						
(first 6 months)		+550	+2.3	46	1 200	10

[1] Energy and Protein Requirements. Report of a Joint FAO/WHO Expert Group, FAO, Rome, 1972. — [2] As egg or milk protein. — [3] Requirements of Vitamin A, Thiamine, Riboflavin and Niacin. Report of a Joint FAO/WHO Export Group, FAO, Rome, 1965. — [4] As retinol. — [5] Requirements of Ascorbic Acid, Vitamin D, Vitamin B_{12}, Folate and Iron. Report of a Joint FAO/WHO Expert Group, FAO, Rome, 1970. — [6] As cholecalciferol. — [7] Calcium Requirements. Report of a FAO/WHO Expert Group, FAO, Rome, 1961. — [8] On each line the lower value applies when over 25 percent of calories in the diet come from animal foods, and the

mine	Ribo-flavine	Niacin	Folic acid	Vitamin B_{12}	Ascorbic acid	Calcium	Iron
3)	(3)	(3)	(5)	(5)	(5)	(7)	(5, 8)
milli-grams	milli-grams	milli-grams	micro-grams	micro-grams	milli-grams	grams	milli-grams
.3	0.5	5.4	60	0.3	20	0.5-0.6	5-10
.5	0.8	9.0	100	0.9	20	0.4-0.5	5-10
.7	1.1	12.1	100	1.5	20	0.4-0.5	5-10
.9	1.3	14.5	100	1.5	20	0.4-0.5	5-10
.0	1.6	17.2	100	2.0	20	0.6-0.7	5-10
.2	1.7	19.1	200	2.0	30	0.6-0.7	9-18
.2	1.8	20.3	200	2.0	30	0.5-0.6	5-9
.9	1.4	15.5	100	2.0	20	0.6-0.7	5-10
.0	1.5	16.4	200	2.0	30	0.6-0.7	12-24
.9	1.4	15.2	200	2.0	30	0.5-0.6	14-28
.2	1.8	19.8	200	2.0	30	0.4-0.5	5-9
.9	1.3	14.5	200	2.0	30	0.4-0.5	14-28
.1	+0.2	+2.3	400	3.0	50	1.0-1.2	(9)
.2	+0.4	+3.7	300	2.5	50	1.0-1.2	(9)

higher value when animal foods represent less than 10 percent of calories. — [9] For women whose iron intake throughout life has been at the level recommended in this table, the daily intake of iron during pregnancy and lactation should be the same as that recommended for nonpregnant, nonlactating women of childbearing age. For women whose iron status is not satisfactory at the beginning of pregnancy, the requirement is increased, and in the extreme situation of women with no iron stores, the requirement can probably not be met without supplementation.

73

TABLE 2. — ENERGY EXPENDITURE OF A 65-KG REFERENCE MAN DISTRIBUTED OVER 24 HOURS AND EFFECT OF OCCUPATION

Distribution of activity	Light activity		Moderately active		Very active		Exceptionally active	
	kilo-calories	mega-joules	kilo-calories	mega-joules	kilo-calories	mega-joules	kilo-calories	mega-joules
In bed (8 hours) . .	500	2.1	500	2.1	500	2.1	500	2.1
At work (8 hours) .	1 100	4.6	1 400	5.8	1 900	8.0	2 400	10.0
Nonoccupational activities	700-	3.0-	700-	3.0-	700-	3.0-	700-	3.0-
(8 hours)	1 500-	6.3-	1 500	6.3	1 500	6.3	1 500	6.3
Range of energy expenditure	2 300-	9.7-	2 600-	10.9-	3 100-	13.0-	3 600-	15.1-
(24 hours).	3 100	13.0	3 400	14.2	3 900	16.3	4 400	18.4
Mean (24 hours) . .	2 700	11.3	3 000	12.5	3 500	14.6	4 000	16.7
Mean (per kg of body weight) . . .	42	0.17	46	0.19	54	0.23	62	0.26

TABLE 3. — ENERGY EXPENDITURE OF A 55-KG REFERENCE WOMAN DISTRIBUTED OVER 24 HOURS AND EFFECT OF OCCUPATION

Distribution of activity	Light activity		Moderately active		Very active		Exceptionally active	
	kilo-calories	mega-joules	kilo-calories	mega-joules	kilo-calories	mega-joules	kilo-calories	mega-joules
In bed (8 hours) . .	420	1.8	420	1.8	420	1.8	420	1.8
At work (8 hours) .	800	3.3	1 000	4.2	1 400	5.9	1 800	7.5
Nonoccupational activities	580-	2.4-	580-	2.4-	580-	2.4-	580-	2.4-
(8 hours)	980	4.1	980	4.1	980	4.1	980	4.1
Range of energy expenditure	1 800-	7.5-	2 000-	8.4-	2 400-	10.1-	2 800-	11.7-
(24 hours).	2 200	9.2	2 400	10.1	2 700	11.8	3 200	13.4
Mean (24 hours) . .	2 000	8.4	2 200	9.2	2 600	10.9	3 000	12.5
Mean (per kg of body weight) . . .	36	0.15	40	0.17	47	0.20	55	0.23

P 335